You and Leukemia

A Day at a Time

Si vous avez un énoncé qui diffère
des renseignements que vous
avez déjà obtenus, veuillez
demander des explications à un
membre de votre équipe de soins
de santé

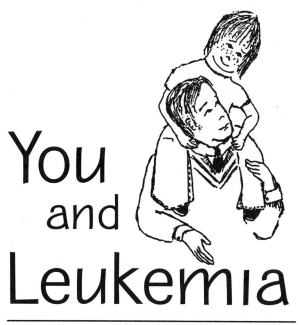

You and Leukemia

A Day at a Time

written and illustrated by

Lynn S. Baker, M.D.

First Edition written in collaboration with

Charles G. Roland, M.D. and Gerald S. Gilchrist, M.D.

W.B. SAUNDERS COMPANY
A Harcourt Health Sciences Company
Philadelphia London Montreal Sydney Tokyo Toronto

W.B. SAUNDERS COMPANY
A Harcourt Health Sciences Company

The Curtis Center
Independence Square West
Philadelphia, Pennsylvania 19106

Acquisition Editor: Elizabeth M. Fathman
Project Manager: Peggy Fagen
Designer: Judi Lang

YOU AND LEUKEMIA: A Day at a Time, 2nd edition   ISBN 0-7216-9067-X

Printed in the United States of America

Last digit is the print number: 9   8   7   6   5   4   3   2   1

❧ Contents ❧

Foreword

This book is literally a handbook on childhood leukemia. It has been especially written so that it can be read by most children over 8 or 9 and understood by children of all ages. The beautiful illustrations can be easily appreciated by preschool children. The book should also provide parents of affected children with many insights into the disease and its management. It answers many of the questions that "we were afraid to ask" or didn't ask because "the doctor seemed to be so busy." Most aspects of the disease and its management are discussed in great depth with the parents at the time of diagnosis and before beginning treatment, but it would be a remarkable parent who was able to comprehend and retain this mass of information in the midst of the emotional upheaval that surrounds these early meetings.

We have long recognized the need for this type of informational material, but it took the interest, insight, and talent of Dr. Baker to bring the idea to fruition. With improvements in the treatment of children with acute leukemia comes an increase in the complexity of the programs. This complexity makes *You and Leukemia* particularly valuable. It is our sincere hope that this book will be made available to every family of every child with leukemia and that it will be a continued source of hope and inspiration to them. It should also prove useful to nurses, social workers, teachers, and all others who have the privilege of working with these children and their families.

The medical community owes a great debt of gratitude to Dr. Baker for her love and devotion in producing this remarkable publication, which was originally developed during an elective rotation in her junior year as a student at Mayo Medical School.

Gerald S. Gilchrist, M.D.
Professor of Pediatrics
Mayo Medical School
Consultant in Pediatric
    Hematology and Oncology
Mayo Clinic & Foundation
Rochester, Minnesota

Charles G. Roland, M.D.
Professor of the History of Medicine
McMaster University
Hamilton, Ontario

with love and good wishes to

Billy

Christine

Cindy

Danny

Greg

Jerilyn

Jody

Kelly

Lana

Lisa

Michael

Tammy

Tanya

Wade

and their families

Preface

This book was written for children with leukemia and for the people who care for and about them. Whichever of these you are, I hope you will find here the knowledge you are seeking. In addition, I hope you will develop a sense of kinship with the many people who have contributed their thoughts, feelings, experience, and time to this project over the years.

Once upon a time, this book was just an idea. I was a medical student at Mayo Medical School with an interest in hematology (diseases of the blood) and in writing, especially for patients. At the time, I was still more patient than doctor myself, and it seemed to me that if I could understand medicine, any-body could. Dr. Charles Roland, then Chairman of the Department of Biomed-ical Communications at Mayo Clinic, and Dr. Gerald Gilchrist, Consultant in Pediatric Hematology and Oncology (cancer) at Mayo Clinic, were my original mentors back in the spring of 1975 when I first set out to write this book.

After that, a whole bunch of people in many different places became part of this book. First, there were Drs. William Krivit, Mark Nesbitt, and Peter Coccia at the University of Minnesota, where I spent several weeks learning how they took care of leukemia patients. It was an exciting time, because the first bone marrow transplants were being done then. After that, I went back to Mayo and worked with Dr. Gilchrist and his colleagues E. Omer Burgert, Jr., and William A. Smithson. Their clinical trials were supported by grants CA04646 and CA15083 from the National Cancer Institute (NCI).

A number of other people at Mayo Clinic contributed to the content of this book, each in his or her own way. They included Carol McCarthy, psychiatric social worker; Barbara Cox, instructional development specialist; Roy Ritts, M.D., immunologist; Ward Fowler, M.D., Dean of Academic Affairs at Mayo Medical School; Rosemary Perry of the Department of Publications; and many residents and interns (physicians-in-training). Once the book was fin-ished, its initial publication and distribution, in 1976, were made possible by John Ivins, M.D., orthopedic oncologist, and his Cancer Rehabilitation Coor-dinating Committee under NCI Contract CN 45120. Kris Gunderson, Bob Denniston, and Cynthia Harryman, all then of the Office of Cancer Communications, also helped by performing what became a very big job— getting the book to the people who needed it.

But within a short time, we ran out of books. At that moment, W.B. Saunders stepped in and rescued *You and Leukemia,* thanks to my then-editor Brian Decker. The new publisher made a commitment to keep the cost of the book as low as possible so that anyone who needed it could afford it—a commit-ment they have kept in the face of rising costs and the highly specialized na-ture of the book.

The first foreign language edition of the book appeared in 1982, with its publication in Japan. Many others have followed, and I have been privileged to hear from patients and families all over the world.

In the mid-eighties, there had been enough advances in the treatment of leukemia that it was time to do a new revision. My partners this time were Jerry Finklestein, M.D., of the UCLA Department of Pediatrics; Joel Cherlow, M.D., radiation oncologist; and Claudia Lee and her staff at the Jonathan Jacques Children's Cancer Center, Memorial Medical Center of Long Beach, California. They not only helped with the new revision but also realized an important dream: the translation and publication of *You and Leukemia* in Spanish.

Now, I am once again revising the book that was only an idea once upon a time. Twenty-five years later so much has changed in the treatment of leukemia—and for the better—that this is truly a happy task. Most impressive is that most children diagnosed with leukemia today will survive their disease. But equally important is the change in the way the medical community approaches the ill child and his or her family. There is a truly cooperative team spirit now. And children's needs are honored. These needs may be physical, such as assuring adequate pain management, or psychological, such as allowing parents to stay overnight in their children's hospital rooms.

The purpose of the original book was not only to provide children and their families with the knowledge they needed to adjust to a devastating illness but also to prepare them for the likelihood of a terrible loss. My purpose now is to prepare most children and families for life with leukemia—and after. Most, but not all. My challenge was to offer very realistic hope while allowing for the fact that there isn't a cure for everyone.

This time around I was again blessed in the help I received. Nancy Baxter of the Leukemia and Lymphoma Society, Greater Los Angeles Chapter, was to become my networking angel. Our meeting at all was a small miracle. My son, Christopher, was dating Nancy's daughter, Rachael. Our two families had dinner together one night. I didn't know what her job was—and Nancy didn't know I had written *You and Leukemia.* Only later did we realize we had another common interest. Without Nancy, I never would have met the rest of the angels who became closely involved with this new edition.

Pauline Hunt, R.N., of Los Angeles Women's and Children's Hospital, was (and is) fantastic. She spent hours of her time both reading several drafts and sitting with me going over them word by word. Marina Perez, B.A., Health Educator at Team CHLA—which is what the Pediatric Oncology team at Children's Hospital of Los Angeles call themselves—hooked me up with all the other members. Besides Marina, all of these generous and expert women reviewed the book: Janet L. Franklin, M.D., pediatric oncologist; Kathy Ruccione, R.N., M.P.H., Center Nursing Administrator; Joyce Derrickson, R.N., radiation oncology; Lisa Bove, L.C.S.W., M. Div., and Lorena Vega, M.S.W., clinical social workers, Leukemia/Lymphoma Program; and Nancy Hart, R.N., and Sherri Carcich, R.N., case managers on the Leukemia/Lymphoma Team.

Thanks, too, go to Carla Arrington, who saved me countless hours by converting the book into a usable computer document—the prior version, naturally, being trapped in a program that no longer exists; to my daughter Cathy, who helped make sure all the illustrations were on the right pages; and to my new editor at Harcourt Health Sciences, Liz Fathman, for her patience when the complexities of life threatened this edition.

Still, and always, the most important people were the patients themselves. It is to them that this book is dedicated and through them that I learned not only what to say but how to say it. If you find on these pages a sense of fun, it is because I was taught that laughter does not end where leukemia begins. These children, and their families, shared their insights, experiences, confusion, pain, observations, discoveries—their lives—with me . . . and so with you. Theirs is a truly special generosity. They were part of this project long before the writing began. They have gone through the book page by page to keep it accurate, interesting, and real. It was they who provided the title and who encouraged its openness and its tone. They are speaking to you on every page.

Lynn S. Baker, M.D.

Introduction

Most books are meant to be read from beginning to end. This book is no different. The reason is that there are many words and ideas you will need to be familiar with in order to understand leukemia. The beginning of this book contains explanations of these words and ideas. If you read this section first, the later sections should not be confusing. Words that are strange at first will seem like old friends by the end.

In case you just want to pick out certain parts to read, we've done two things. If you find a word that is unfamiliar to you, you can turn to the index at the very back of the book and look for the word there. The page where the word is defined will be listed, and you can look it up in the text. We've also made a glossary of words that are not defined in the text. You can find this in the back of the book as well, right before the index. Both the index and the glossary contain keys for pronouncing the words, so you can sound just like your doctors and nurses when you say them.

There are some other sections in the last half of the book that are important. The longest is the special section on Treatment that begins on page 136. In the text we talk in general terms about treatment, but we don't go into much detail because the details can seem overwhelming at first. But after a while you'll have a lot of questions about treatment, and this section should answer most of them. There is also a list of additional resources you can turn to if you want to learn more about the body, medicine, and leukemia.

One group of people may have some trouble reading this book—the patients. Many of you are very young and haven't had a lot of experience reading. We hope you can find someone who is a good reader to help you (and maybe your brothers and sisters) learn about leukemia. If you're under ten years old, you'll probably need some help, but we think the person who helps you will be surprised at how well you'll be able to understand it. After all, it's about you. That means it's really interesting. And remember, as you get older, you'll be able to read it by yourself.

You will notice that there are some blank pages in the book. These are for you and your family to fill in with the help of your doctors and nurses. We hope you will feel free to use these pages. We want the book to grow with you, to be used in any way you wish. Whatever you want to do—color the pictures, glue in photographs, write your own thoughts, save magazine and newspaper articles—do it. That's what it's for.

We who worked on this book over the years hope you will find it useful. It will always be there to answer your questions. It will never be "too busy." Of course, it will never be able to answer *all* your questions—no one book can.

We hope too that you will talk to each other, and to your doctors and nurses, about the things in this book. The more we all know about leukemia, the better we will all be able to live with it, each in our own way. Finally, I hope that you will feel free to share your ideas with me. I don't know what the next 25 years will bring, but based on the last quarter century there are sure to be even more advances in the treatment of leukemia and this book will need to be revised again. That means your ideas are important. You can e-mail me at lsbmdwords@aol.com

Lynn S. Baker, M.D.

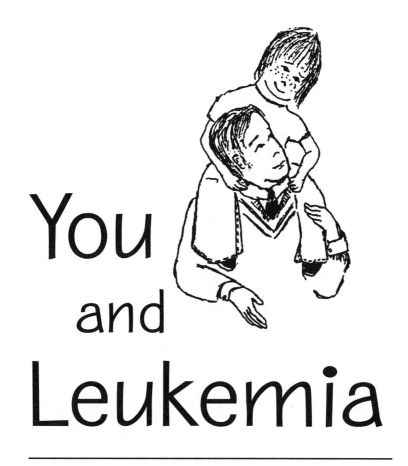

You
and
Leukemia

A Day at a Time

You . . .

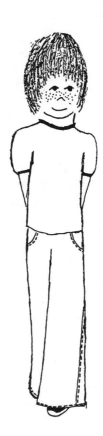

You

are very special.

That's why this book was written:

for you.

about you.

And since you are the most

important person

in the book.

this page is for your picture

and your name.

My name is

_____

and this is my book.

You are a person.

All people are like each other in some ways

and not alike in others.

This book was made for you by other people.

Some of them are children, like you,

who have leukemia too.

They want to tell you about having leukemia

so that you will know what they have learned.

Some of them are parents or doctors or nurses

or friends, like yours.

They want to tell you what they have learned too.

They think that if you know about leukemia,

it won't be so strange to you.

And when things are not so strange

they are not so scary.

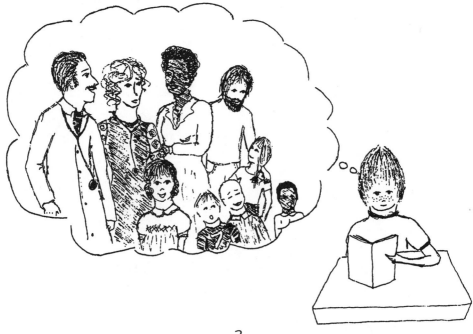

Leukemia is a strange disease.

Not even doctors know all about it yet.

This book will tell you what is known now.

Leukemia can't be explained in just a few pages.

In fact, before we can even start

to talk about leukemia,

you have to know a lot of other things.

First, you have to know a little about your body.

And you need to know a lot about blood.

After you have learned about those things

we will talk about leukemia:

about what it is,

about what might cause it,

about how doctors found out you had it,

about what will be done to try to make you better.

At the very end of this book we will talk about you again

about you and your life with leukemia.

And after leukemia.

★Your Body

Part of being you is being your body.

Does that sound funny?

What do you know about your body?

When you look at it, what do you see?

Skin and hair and freckles?

Arms and legs and a belly button?

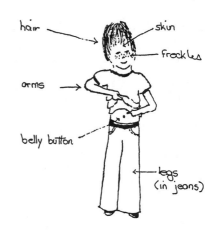

When you look at your body,

you only see part of it—

just the outside covering.

There is an old saying that goes,

"Beauty is only skin deep."

Whoever said that must not have looked.

The part of your body that is under your skin

is as beautiful as anything can be.

Human beings are very lucky.

Not only are we bodies—

we are whole beings,

and we are able to enjoy how beautiful we all are.

Inside and out.

What do you think the inside of your body is like?

If you could unzip your skin and take it off,

like clothes, what would you find?

A whole new world—that's what you'd find.

It's hard to make sense of new worlds at first.

A long time ago, when doctors were learning

about what all those things are in there (anatomy),

what they do (physiology),

and what can go wrong with them (pathology),

doctors got mixed up all the time.

But after a while they began to figure it out.

By the end of this part of the book

you will know more about your body

than the greatest scientist did 200 years ago.

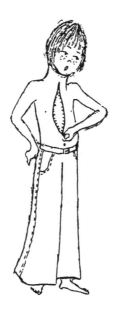

⬦Cells

If we are going to do this right we'd best

start at the beginning: the cell.

A cell is the smallest bit of you that is still

definitely you—and no one else.

Here is a picture of a cell.

You probably won't think it looks much like you.

That's because you are made of millions of

different kinds of cells.

But once upon a time you were just one cell,

and you didn't look much like you then, either.

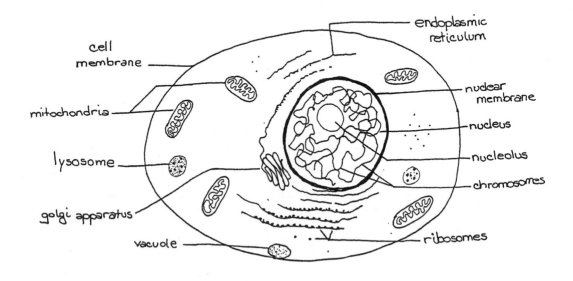

That one cell that was you

had a plan in its nucleus (its brain).

It divided again and again

following that plan.

Some of its great-grandchildren

became liver cells

and others became skin cells,

all according to the plan

to make you.

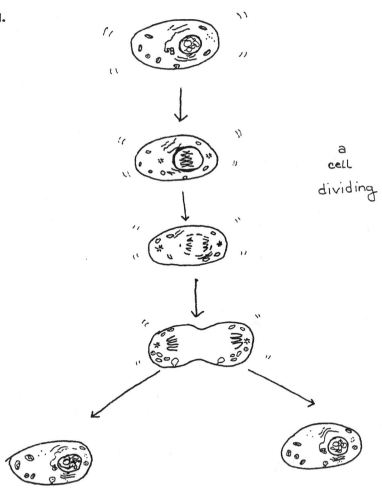

a
cell
dividing

All of your millions of cells,

no matter how different they might seem,

still have that same plan in their nucleus.

Each part of the plan is called a gene.

See the strings in the nucleus picture?

They are called chromosomes.

Chromosomes are made of many genes

all in a row.

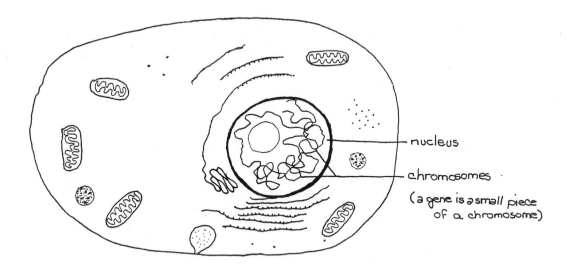

nucleus

chromosomes

(a gene is a small piece
of a chromosome)

Your genes (and so your chromosomes)

are made of long stringy molecules

called DNA.

The plan to make you

is your DNA.

You are you because your DNA is put together

in a very special way.

If your DNA had been put together differently,

you might have been a giraffe or a tuna fish.

You are the only living being in the whole world

whose cells contain your genes, your DNA.

This is important and we will be talking about it again.

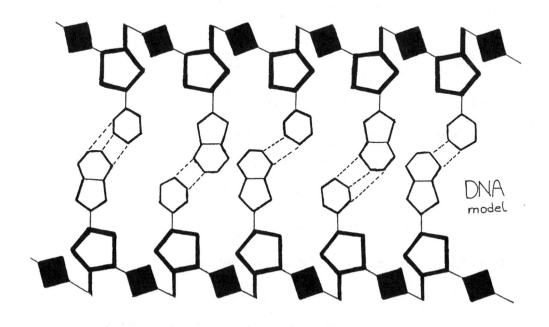

DNA
model

❖Organs and Organ Systems

Your body is made up of millions of cells

the same way a big city is made up of millions of people.

Like people in a city, each of your cells has a job to do.

When many cells all do the same job

and they don't have to move around much to do it,

they gather in one place and work together.

The group of cells is then called an organ.

In a city, people who all do the same job organize, too.

They might all go to the same place to work

or they might get together in labor unions.

People—and cells—often get jobs done better

when they work together.

When there is a really big job to be done,

organs get together and work with other organs.

Each organ will do a part of the work.

When organs work together like this,

they are called an organ system.

In a city, the same kind of thing happens.

Hospitals, doctors, nurses, and ambulances

are all parts of the health care system.

Each group does a different part of the work for that one system.

Groups of people—like organs—often get jobs done better

when they work together.

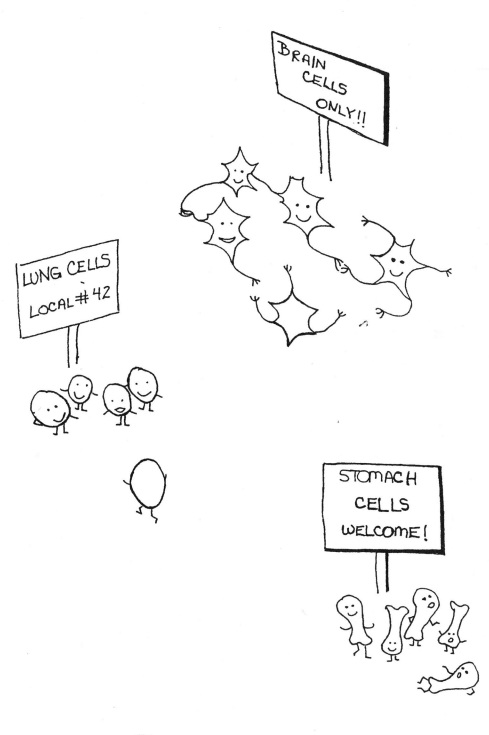

Your body has many organs and several systems.

These systems work to keep you going

the same way that people, groups of people and systems

work to keep a city going.

What sorts of systems do you think your body—

or a city—might need?

Well, first of all, you need food and so do cities.

That is what your digestive system is for.

The digestive system is your body's grocery store.

Every time you eat, your digestive system works hard

to break up the food into pieces that are little enough

for your cells to use them to get energy.

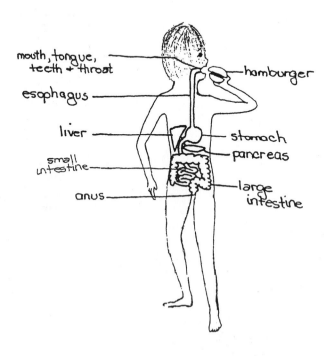

You need something else to get energy out of food.

You need oxygen—air—and so do cities.

That is what your respiratory system is for.

The respiratory system is your body's oxygen supplier.

Your cells use oxygen to help them burn up your food

faster and better—

the same way that charcoal lighter fluid helps you burn

charcoal faster and better.

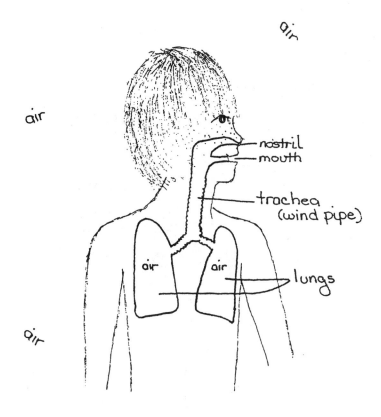

Cities have factories, and so do you.

One group of factories is called the endocrine system.

These factories, called glands, all make hormones.

Hormones are chemicals your entire body needs

to grow right and feel good.

Other factories are parts of other systems.

They make things that those systems need

to do their work right.

Some of the organs of your digestive system, for example,

make chemicals to help break food up into little pieces.

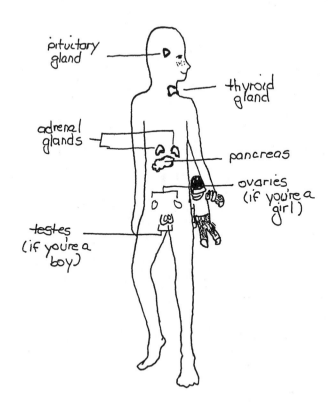

Now, we know that burning things,

making energy and running factories

all cause pollution in cities.

Your body is no different.

It needs a system to get rid of wastes

and recycle the good stuff.

This is what the excretory system does.

It is your body's recycling center.

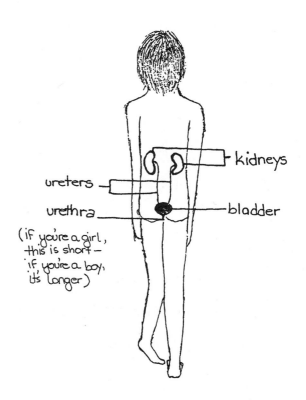

kidneys

ureters

urethra

bladder

(if you're a girl,
this is short –
if you're a boy,
it's longer)

Cities have downtowns with neighborhoods around them.

Your downtown is your chest and belly

where all of the systems we've talked about are found.

The neighborhoods are your bones and muscles,

which are all around you.

They are another system.

They use a lot of your food and oxygen

and make you able to stand and move around

without having to change your shape

(the way a worm has to change its shape

when it moves).

Your skin is another organ system.

It is like the walls that used to be built

around cities in olden times.

It keeps the inside of you inside you

and the outside of you outside you.

It helps to keep your body at the right temperature

by sweating when you are too hot

and getting "goose bumps" when you are too cold.

It helps to keep germs out.

Your skin and muscles and bones together

make up your city's skyline.

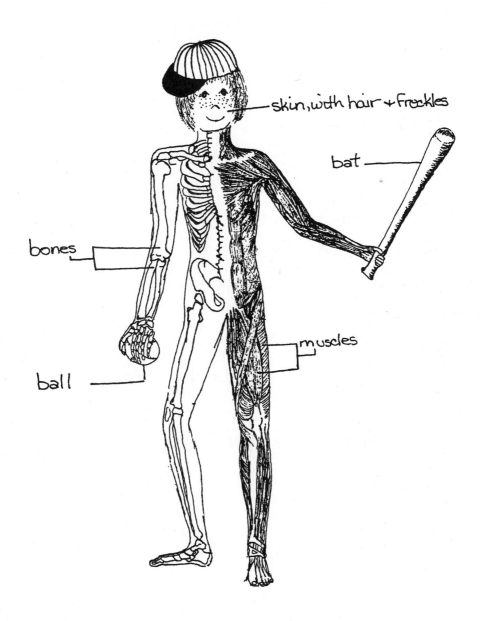

skin, with hair & freckles

bat

bones

ball

muscles

Now, when you've got all of these different cells

and organ systems, and they are all spread out

like a city,

there has to be some kind of government

to keep things working together.

This is what your nervous system is for.

Your brain is your body's mayor.

It figures out what is going on and what needs to be done

with advice from the rest of your body.

Your brain cells can "talk" with other cells

because you have telephone lines, too.

Your nerves are your body's telephone lines.

They are all over your body

the way telephone lines are all over a city.

They let the brain know what's going on far away.

They let your cells and organs know

what the brain wants them to do.

It's a two-way thing.

It is in cities, too.

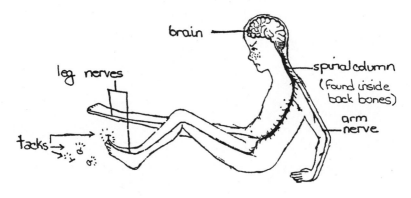

Cities need a system of roads, too.

How else can things get from the factories

to the people who need them?

How else can food get from the grocery stores

to your table?

Your body has two kinds of roads:

the blood vessels and the lymphatic vessels.

They are like little tubes

and they make up your circulatory system.

They go to every cell in your body

the way roads connect every building in a city.

The engine that drives or pushes the traveler

on the roads is your heart.

There are two kinds of blood vessels.

One kind, the arteries, leads away from the heart.

The other kind, the veins, leads back to the heart.

Lymphatic vessels go in only one direction,

back to the heart.

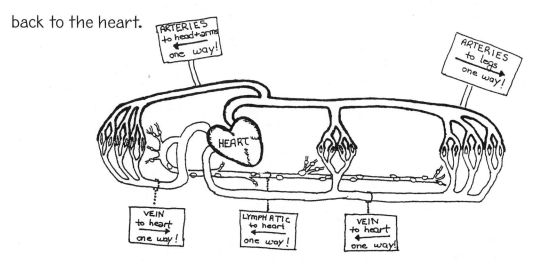

The traveler, of course, is your blood.

If you push gently down

on the inside of your wrist

below your thumb,

you can feel your blood being pushed

through an artery by your heart.

This is your pulse.

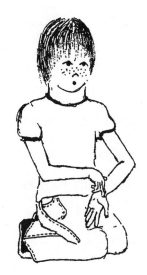

You will learn about blood in the next section.

But now that you know more about your body—

about how nicely it's organized

and how well it works—

could you ever think that beauty is only skin deep?

★ Your Blood

What do you think blood is?

What does it look like?

It looks like a red liquid.

It runs out like water if you get a bad cut,

no matter where you get the cut.

Blood seems to be a red liquid

that is all through your body.

Not quite.

Blood might <u>look</u> like a red liquid

but it isn't.

What blood really is

is a pale, golden, clear liquid

with many tiny cells in it.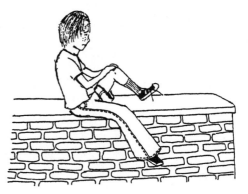

They are called red blood cells

(or RBCs or erythrocytes).

They are why your blood looks red.

If that doesn't make sense,

here is an experiment that you can do.

Pour some tomato juice into a glass.

Put it into the refrigerator

and leave it there for a few days.

Then look at it.

What did it look like when you put it in?

What does it look like now?

See how it is reddest at the bottom

and pale, clear, and golden at the top.

That is because tomato juice

is made up of tiny bits of tomatoes

and golden juice.

When it's all mixed up,

it looks like a red liquid.

But it really isn't.

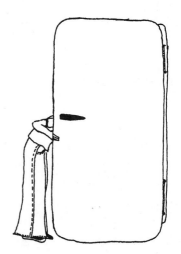

Not all of the cells in your blood are red.

Some are white—well, they are really almost clear

but we call them white.

These are the white blood cells

(or WBCs or leukocytes).

There are also many very teeny cells

called platelets

(or thrombocytes).

The pale, clear, golden liquid

is called plasma

(it doesn't have any other names).

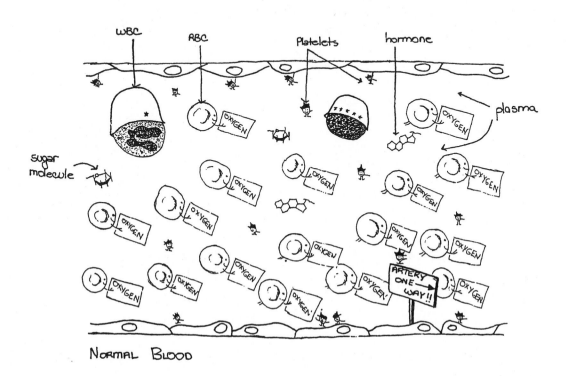

Normal Blood

◇What Does Blood Do?

Let's pretend that your body is a city
with all the different parts you already know about in it.
Your factories, grocery store and oxygen supplier
need something to carry the things they make or have
to all the rest of your cells.
You need something to carry wastes
to your recycling center.
This is part of what blood does.

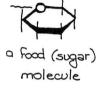

a food (sugar)
molecule

The food you eat is carried in the plasma
to every part of your city.
The things the factories make—like hormones—
are carried in the plasma, too.

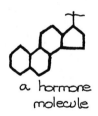

a hormone
molecule

The oxygen in the air you breathe
is carried by the red blood cells (RBCs)
to all parts of your city.
RBCs are the body's delivery trucks.

All cities need policemen to keep the trucks on the road.
This is what platelets do.
Platelets are the blood's policemen.
They have helpers in the plasma, and they work together
to keep your blood inside your blood vessels.

Sometimes cities need armies, too, to defend them from nasty outsiders.

This is what the white blood cells (WBCs) do.

WBCs are the body's soldiers.

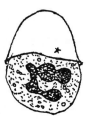

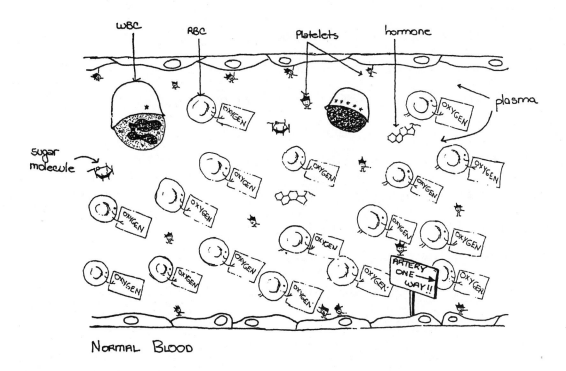

NORMAL BLOOD

Now we can learn more about what blood does.

Let's pretend that your city doesn't have
enough delivery trucks (RBCs).
What would happen?
Well, for one thing, your blood wouldn't be so red.
That would make you pale.
For another, your cells wouldn't get
all the oxygen that they need.
That would make you tired and weak.
You would breathe very hard to get more air.
But without enough RBCs to carry the oxygen,
no matter how hard you breathe
your cells still won't get enough.
Your heart will work very hard
to make the blood go around faster.
That helps, but it makes you more tired.
Your heart works so hard that it sometimes
begins to complain.
As the blood goes through it, it makes a noise
called a murmur.
But that doesn't mean that there's anything wrong
with the heart itself.

When there aren't enough red cells—

or when something is wrong with them

and they can't do their job—

you have anemia.

There are many different causes of anemia.

Leukemia is one of them.

But no matter what causes the anemia,

the result is always the same.

You get pale, tired and weak.

You might get a heart murmur.

You might get so that you don't care about much.

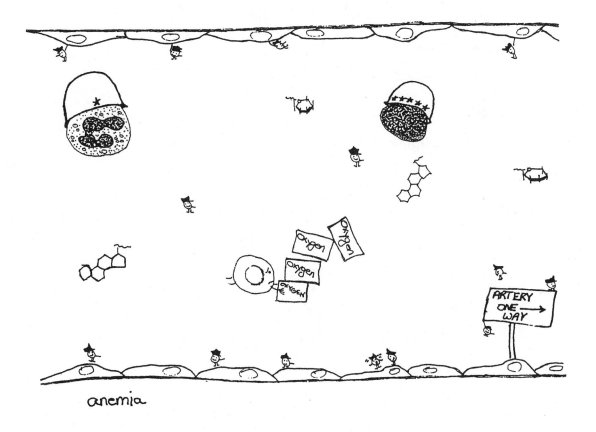

anemia

Now let's pretend something else.

Let's pretend that your red cells are OK,

only now your city doesn't have

enough police officers (platelets).

What do you think might happen?

Well, for one thing,

what if you cut your finger?

Usually when you do that,

it bleeds for a while and then stops.

It is the platelets and their helpers in the plasma

that make it stop.

They get sticky and make a plug in the hole.

They keep blood inside the blood vessels,

where it's supposed to be.

Without platelets, you will bleed longer.

You can bleed inside your skin, too.

That is what a bruise is.

Without platelets, you get bruises more easily

and more often, and they are bigger than they should be.

You can bleed for almost no reason at all.

You may suddenly start to bleed from your gums or nose.

Or your tiniest blood vessels can leak

and you might get little red spots,

like freckles, on your skin.

These are called petechiae.

When you don't have enough platelets,

you have thrombocytopenia.

There are many different causes of thrombocytopenia.

Leukemia is one of them.

But no matter what causes thrombocytopenia,

the result is always the same.

You bleed longer.

You bruise easier.

You can bleed from your gums or nose.

You might get petechiae.

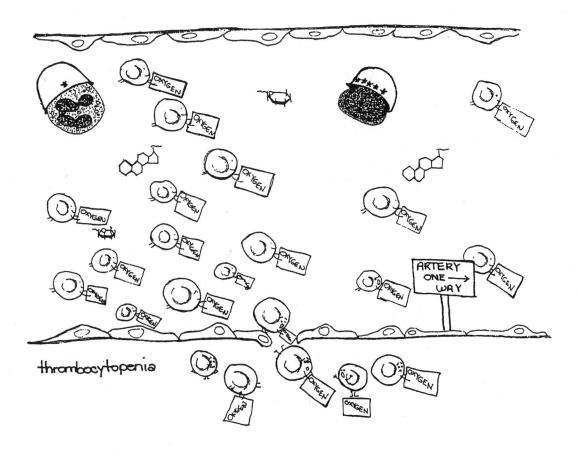

thrombocytopenia

Let's pretend something else.

Let's pretend that your city has enough RBCs and platelets,

but there aren't enough soldiers (WBCs).

What do you think might happen?

What if your city was invaded by an army of nasty germs?

Usually, your WBCs get together and fight them off.

There is more than one kind of WBC,

and each one fights your enemies

in its own way.

A soldier in the army fights enemies on land.

A sailor in the navy fights enemies on the sea.

But both of them fight enemies.

They might even fight the same enemy in different ways.

That is the way it is with WBCs.

Without them, the germs can do whatever they want.

They can steal your food and your oxygen.

They can close down the factories.

They can tangle up the telephone lines

and mix up your mayor.

If your city can't defend itself,

it's in serious trouble.

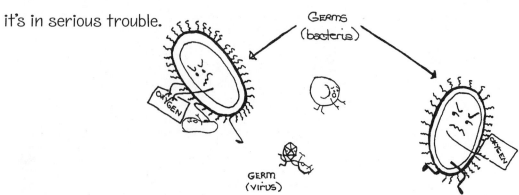

Germs
(bacteria)

Oxygen

Germ
(virus)

When you don't have enough

of all of the different kinds of WBCs,

you have leukopenia.

There are many causes of leukopenia.

The drugs that are used to treat leukemia

can be one cause.

But no matter what causes the leukopenia,

the result is always the same.

Your body will not be able to defend itself,

you may get more infections

and these infections could be more serious.

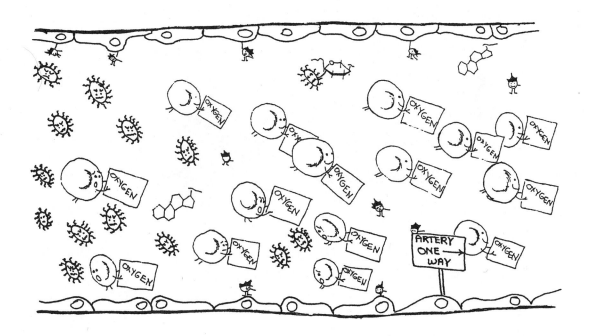

So far it's all been pretty simple.

But because there is more than one kind of WBC,

now it gets a little more complicated.

Since WBCs are what leukemia is all about,

you have to know a lot more about them.

One kind of WBC

is called a granulocyte.

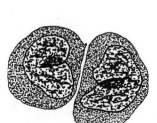

It is the best soldier you have

for fighting the group of germs called bacteria

and the diseases they cause—like strep throat.

Granulocytes fight bacteria

by surrounding them—and then eating them!

Granulocytes are best at "search and destroy" jobs.

A second kind of WBC

is called a monocyte.

It will fight any kind of germ

anywhere in your body.

It kills germs by eating them too.

But monocytes aren't as picky as granulocytes.

They'll eat anything!

Monocytes are your body's guerilla soldiers.

The last kind of WBC is called a lymphocyte.

There are two kinds of lymphocytes.

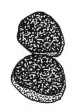

B-lymphocytes have a special job.

They spray germs—or anything else they find inside you

that they don't think should be there—

with sticky stuff called antibodies.

Antibodies are like signs that tell other WBCs,

"This is an enemy. Get it!"

Those signs really help other WBCs do their jobs.

B-lymphocytes are best at being scouts.

T-lymphocytes do both commanding and fighting.

They send chemical orders to other WBCs:

"Here's where the trouble is. Get here right away!"

When the other WBCs get to where the trouble is,

T-lymphocytes make sure they stay there.

These cells can also help brand-new WBCs

do their jobs like old pros.

They give chemical commands that tell other lymphocytes

to divide and make even more lymphocytes.

There are even some T-lymphocytes that tell other WBCs

to <u>stop</u> fighting when fighting is no longer necessary.

T-lymphocytes give lots of orders, but they are soldiers, too,

especially against germs like viruses and funguses.

T-lymphocytes are your body's field commanders.

So, you can see that you need enough

of all kinds of WBCs

to defend yourself against all kinds of germs.

If one kind is missing, you could still defend yourself,

but not as well.

All of your WBCs must be there,

must do their work right

and must do it together

for you to stay healthy.

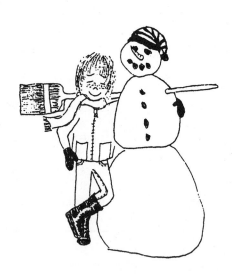

What does blood do?

It keeps you going.

It makes sure that all of you has

> food

> air

> water

And it keeps trouble-makers away.

Red juice?

It looks like that,

but it's much more wonderful.

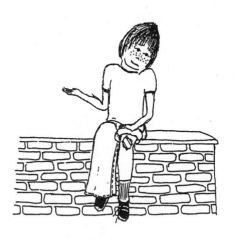

❖Where Is Blood Made?

Blood cells are made in your bones.

Does that surprise you?

You know that bones hold you up

and protect your squishy parts.

But they also make blood cells.

Deep inside each bone,

protected by the hard part,

is the bone marrow.

This is another of your body's factories.

All types of blood cells are made here.

All blood cells, no matter what kind they are,

seem to start out as a single, special kind of cell—

the stem cell.

A stem cell can become

(depending on what the body needs)

a red cell or a white cell

or a cell that makes platelets.

Amazing.

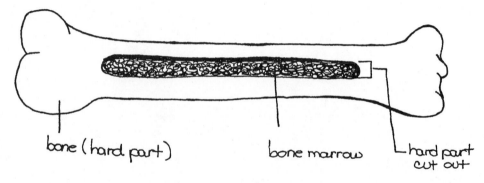

bone (hard part)   bone marrow   hard part cut out

But you are like a stem cell in some ways.

You might grow up to be a police officer (platelet)

or a soldier (WBC)

or a delivery-truck driver (RBC).

What's more, even if you grow up to be a soldier,

you might have a baby who grows up to be a police officer.

Stem cells do that, too.

They make new stem cells,

besides growing up to be more specialized cells.

Stem cells are amazing.

And so are you.

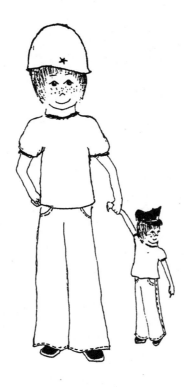

Now, let's say that you decide you want to be a soldier.

There's a lot you have to do before you can be one.

You have to get older, bigger, stronger.

That takes time.

You have to finish school.

You have to get special training.

There are many stages that you must go through

before you can be a soldier.

If a stem cell is going to be a WBC (or an RBC or a platelet),

it also has to go through certain stages.

Each stage has a name,

like "high school graduate" or "new recruit."

Only, for each kind of cell, there are different names.

You will learn these names later.

The whole growth process is called maturation,

and it happens in the bone marrow for most blood cells.

Some young lymphocytes may move to a lymph node,

or the thymus gland or the spleen

to grow up, live, work

and make new lymphocytes.

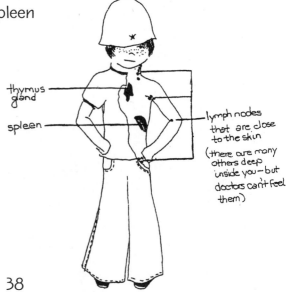

thymus gland

spleen

lymph nodes that are close to the skin

(there are many others deep inside you — but doctors can't feel them)

Usually, a cell won't leave its growing-up place

until it is all done growing up.

Usually, but not always.

When something goes wrong, immature cells

(cells that haven't grown up yet) may be sent out.

When a doctor sees immature cells in your blood,

he or she knows that all is not well.

Sending an immature cell out into the blood

would be like sending you out to be a soldier

without letting you grow up and learn how first.

You wouldn't be able to do the job very well.

Understanding bone marrow is very important

in understanding blood.

Bone marrow is where blood cells are born and raised.

Anything that goes wrong in the bone marrow

will show up as something wrong in the blood,

eventually.

Anything that goes wrong in the blood

will show up as something wrong with you,

eventually.

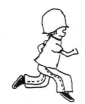

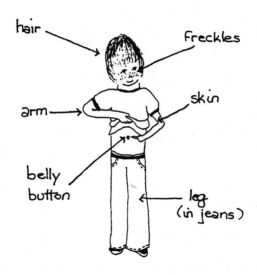

hair

freckles

arm

skin

belly
button

leg
(in jeans)

...and
Leukemia

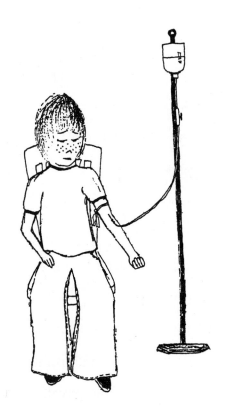

★ What Is Leukemia?

It is easy to answer that question.

The problem is in understanding the answer.

Leukemia is a cancer of the white blood cells.

Cancer is when a bunch of cells

won't work with the rest of your body.

They get selfish.

They won't follow the rules.

They divide when they feel like it,

which usually isn't when they're supposed to.

They don't do their work right (if they do it at all).

They crowd out normal cells,

so the normal cells can't work right either.

Cancer cells don't stay in the organ they belong to.

They travel all over the body

and stop wherever they like.

They probably don't mean to cause trouble

but they do, and for this reason

they are called "malignant."

Any cell in your body can become malignant.

If the white blood cells become malignant,

the disease is called leukemia.

malignant cells   normal cells

★ What Causes Leukemia?

No one can answer this question.

Many people are working hard to find the answer.

If they do, you will be told about it.

But there is no exact answer now.

Several possibilities are being studied, however.

These possible causes will be listed in this section.

But before they are listed, there is something you should know.

You or a member of your family or a friend,

may be feeling guilty because you have leukemia.

Maybe you're afraid that something you did

might have caused it.

Maybe you think that your leukemia

is a punishment for something.

That if you, or they, are "bad," you might get sicker.

It is important to remember, and to remind others,

that as of this time:

∞ Nobody caused your leukemia,

nobody could have prevented it.

The possible causes or contributing factors
are usually divided into three groups:

1. genetic factors (something you're born with)
2. environmental factors (coming from your surroundings)
3. immunologic factors (a problem with your body's ability to
    defend itself)

A FAMILY TREE
(one of the tools scientists use to study genetic factors)

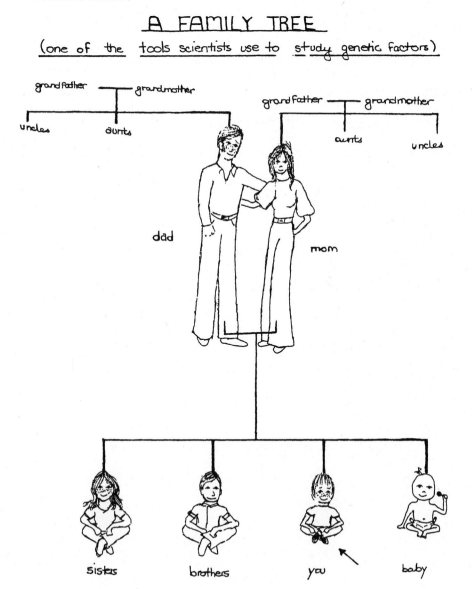

◆Genetic Factors (see pages 6-9)

In each of your cells you have 46 chromosomes.

On these chromosomes, you have millions of genes.

You inherited your genes from your mom and dad,

which is why you're kind of like both of them

but not the same as either of them.

No two people have exactly the same genes except identical twins.

One clue that genes may play a part in causing leukemia

is that when one identical twin gets leukemia,

the second twin is more likely to also get it

than if they were not identical twins.

(But most of the time, the second twin doesn't get it.)

Another clue is that people with unusual chromosomes

get leukemia more often than would be expected.

They might have an extra chromosome, or not enough.

Or their chromosomes are weak and fall apart easily.

But how could a gene, or an abnormal chromosome,

cause leukemia (or any other cancer)?

It turns out that our cells have certain genes

that tell the cell things like "Divide" or "Don't divide anymore."

If one of these genes gets hurt,

it can turn into something called an "oncogene."

An oncogene tells the cell to do the wrong thing,

like to divide when it shouldn't.

Does this sound familiar?

◇Environmental Factors

Things that might turn your normal genes into oncogenes

exist in your environment,

in the world around you.

All of these environmental factors have one thing in common:

they can change the structure of DNA.

DNA is what your genes are made of.

DNA contains the plan to make you

and the rules your cells live by.

There are things in the environment that can change DNA,

so they can probably change the rules.

And, as you know,

malignant cells follow their own rules.

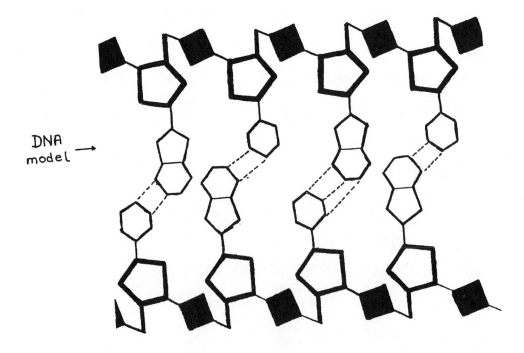

DNA model →

1. Radiation

Radiation is everywhere.

Most of it comes from the sun, and without the sun

there would be no life on our lively planet Earth.

But certain kinds of radiation

can hurt DNA and break chromosomes.

People who have had large amounts of radiation

(really huge amounts, like in a nuclear explosion)

get leukemia more often than other people.

The small amounts of radiation used to take x-rays

don't seem to cause leukemia in anyone.

Larger amounts of radiation, such as that used in radiation therapy,

may cause some people to get leukemia or other cancers

later in life.

X-rays and radiation therapy have helped many people,

including you.

But, just in case, doctors don't

take x-rays of people

without a good reason—

and, just in case, radiation therapy

is never used

unless it's really needed.

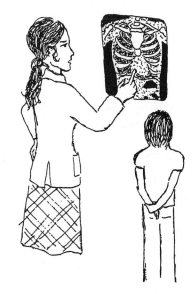

2. Chemicals

Chemicals are everywhere

and there's nothing bad about most of them.

Water is a chemical.

So is spaghetti.

And you are made of zillions of chemicals.

But some chemicals are called "toxic,"

which means they are not good for living things.

Some of these toxic chemicals can hurt DNA and chromosomes.

And some of these, like the ones in tobacco smoke

or a chemical called benzene,

can cause cancer.

But no one has ever found, for sure,

a toxic chemical that causes leukemia.

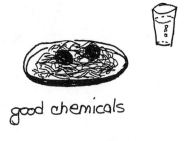

good chemicals

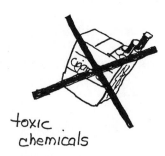

toxic
chemicals

Rarely, a person exposed to one of these chemicals
may get a disease called "aplastic anemia."
In this disease, the bone marrow totally stops working
and no blood cells are made at all.
Sometimes, if the bone marrow starts working again,
it will make leukemia cells instead of normal ones.

Most people who are exposed to these chemicals
don't get either leukemia or aplastic anemia.
Even so, it happens often enough
that some scientists are studying these chemicals
to learn exactly what they do to cells.
And other scientists are trying to find ways
to get rid of these toxic chemicals safely.
People, factories and governments are working together
to make sure no one is exposed to toxic chemicals accidentally.

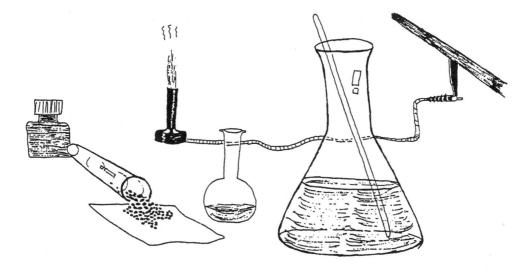

3. Electromagnetic fields

Electricity is all around us.

Lightning is electricity.

You can't play video games without electricity.

There are cars that run on electricity instead of gasoline,

which is a good idea because burning gasoline

makes toxic chemicals.

Magnetic fields are all around us, too.

There are teeny ones around each of your refrigerator magnets.

There are huge ones at both the North and the South Poles

(that's how your compass knows which way to point).

Electromagnetic fields (EMFs) are a combination of the two.

They happen around any electric wire.

There are teeny EMFs around the wire that plugs in your TV.

There are huge EMFs around big bunches of high-power wires

like the ones near power plants.

Scientists are having a big argument about whether or not

these great big EMFs might have something to do

with causing leukemia or other cancers.

No one has won the argument yet,

so no one can say for sure.

But scientists are working together

to try to figure it out.

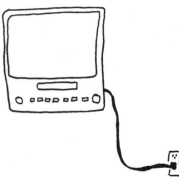

4. Viruses

Viruses are kinds of germs

and they cause lots of different diseases.

Some viruses cause colds and flu.

Others cause warts or chicken pox.

For a long time, scientists have wondered if viruses

might help cause leukemia—and other cancers.

Scientists have found viruses that cause leukemia in animals:

in cows, cats, birds and mice.

But finding viruses that cause, or help to cause,

leukemia in people hasn't been so easy.

Recently, two viruses have been found

that can cause very uncommon forms

of leukemia in grownups.

But no one has found a virus that causes

the more common types of leukemia,

including the ones that happen to children.

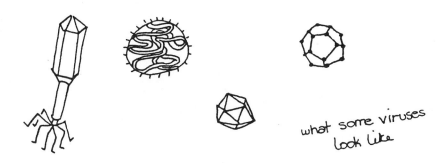

what some viruses
look like

There is a virus called EBV

that may help cause a type of lymphoma

in children who live in Africa.

(The lymphomas are sort of cousins to the leukemias,

but they start out in lymph nodes instead of in bone marrow.)

This lymphoma, called Burkitt's lymphoma,

acts a lot like an infection in Africa.

But many children in Africa

get lots of other infections besides EBV.

Maybe having to fight so many infections

makes these children's immune systems all tired out

and that is why EBV can cause lymphoma in these children.

Maybe, but no one knows.

Besides, there are children who don't live in Africa

or who have never had EBV

who have also gotten this type of lymphoma.

And most children (and grownups) who get EBV

never get lymphoma.

Or leukemia.

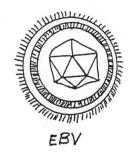

EBV

Other viruses besides EBV have been found in cells

from people with other kinds of cancer.

For example, there are a couple of viruses

that are strongly suspected to help cause liver cancer.

The trouble is, no one knows if those viruses

caused the cancer,

helped to cause the cancer—

or just happened to be there.

One thing scientists do know is that

the way viruses cause diseases

is by putting their own genes,

their own DNA (or something like it called RNA),

into our cells.

And that the viral genes change what our cells do.

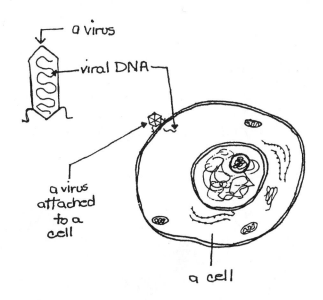

◇Immunologic Factors

You should know about immunologic factors, too.

Immunologic factors (including your WBCs)

help your body defend itself from harm.

They are the subject of an exciting field called immunology.

Scientists and doctors in this field

are trying to answer questions like these:

Why do people get sick at some times and not at others?

Why do some of us get leukemia, but most do not?

Do people with leukemia

have something wrong with their bodies' defenses?

Was the "something wrong" always there

and that's how the leukemia got going?

Or does leukemia itself cause the "something" to go "wrong"?

No one knows yet,

but it makes good sense to ask these kinds of questions.

Even now, immunologists are finding new kinds of treatments

(immunotherapy) that help the body defend itself better.

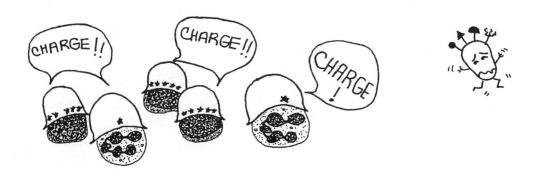

All over the world, people are working to find the factor,

or, more likely, the combination of factors,

that causes leukemia.

They're working for you.

And let's hope, when the cause is found,

that it will be possible to find a cure

or a way to prevent leukemia.

Please remember, though,

what was said at the beginning of this section:

☞ <u>Nobody caused your leukemia,</u>

   <u>nobody could have prevented it.</u>

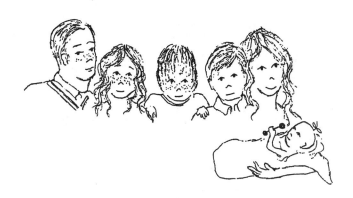

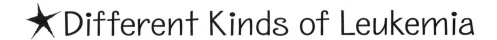Different Kinds of Leukemia

Leukemia is not just one disease.

Since there is more than one kind of WBC,

there has to be more than one kind of leukemia—

in fact, one for each kind of WBC.

This chart shows the different kinds.

LEUKEMIA	
Lymphocytic	Nonlymphocytic
B-cell lineage undifferentiated T-cell lineage	myelogenous (granulocytic) monocytic myelomonocytic progranulocytic erythroleukemia

The most common kinds are

lymphocytic and myelogenous (granulocytic) leukemia.

The other types are very rare.

The rare kinds act a lot like the more common kinds.

And doctors treat them the same way.

If these leukemias affect you quickly, they are "acute."

If they affect you slowly, they are "chronic."

These are old names but they are still used,

so you should know what they mean.

This book is mostly about the acute leukemias.

◈Acute Lymphocytic Leukemia

This is commonly known as "childhood leukemia"

and is referred to as ALL.

It can also be called "acute lymphoblastic leukemia."

Most of the people who get ALL are between two and eight

years old when the disease is diagnosed.

They can be older than that, though, or younger.

More boys get ALL than girls,

but not very many more.

White children get ALL more often

than African-American children.

No one knows why these things are true.

The malignant cell in ALL is an abnormal lymphocyte

called a "lymphoblast" ("blast" for short)

or a "leukemia cell."

It isn't a normal immature lymphocyte.

In most cases, it's a little more like a B-lymphocyte

than it is like a T-lymphocyte (page 33).

But in some cases it's not like either one of them.

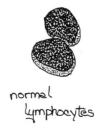

normal
lymphocytes

The blast seems to cause trouble mainly by

crowding the bone marrow

so the normal cells have a hard time growing.

The blasts don't kill the normal cells.

They just get in the way.

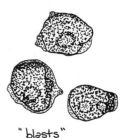

"blasts"

What the blasts do is something like this.

Imagine that you and your family are at home

living your normal lives.

One day a little rabbit walks in the front door and won't leave.

That doesn't upset your lives too much.

But then a few more rabbits show up.

Then more and more, until the whole house

is full of rabbits.

Now that's a problem.

It would be really hard to live a normal life

with rabbits all over the place.

They would cause trouble just by being there.

That's what leukemic blasts do.

They start out in your bone marrow and they fill that up.

But then they go other places, too.

They can go to your lymph nodes

or to your spleen or to your liver.

Actually, they can go anywhere blood goes—

and that's everywhere.

Just as if the rabbits were not only in

your house

but in every building and street in

your city.

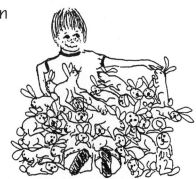

Blasts also cause trouble

by forgetting to grow up.

They stay immature

and keep dividing when they shouldn't.

Because they are so immature,

they can't do their work.

They don't know how to be soldiers.

When trouble comes, they don't give any orders

or do any fighting.

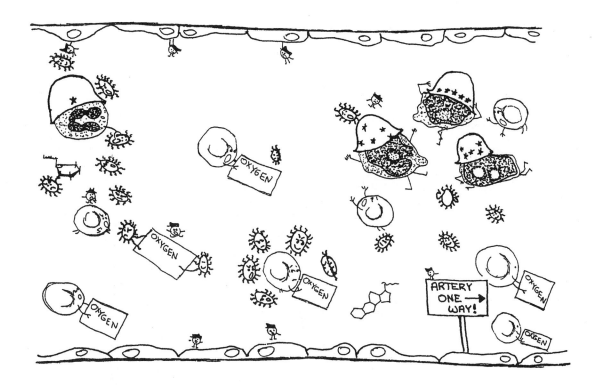

◇Acute Myelogenous Leukemia

This is sometimes referred to as AML

and is also called acute granulocytic leukemia.

It's a disease that usually happens to people over 25.

However, it can happen to teenagers and children.

The malignant cell in AML is an immature granulocyte

called a myeloblast ("blast" for short).

It is also called a leukemia cell, sometimes.

This blast is different from the lymphoblast in ALL,

but it can cause the same kinds of problems.

This disease isn't as easy to understand as ALL,

and it's more difficult to treat.

But doctors all over the world

are sharing their knowledge about AML with each other.

They are trying different ways to treat it

to try to find the best way.

If you have AML,

much of this book will still be helpful to you.

AML is not the same disease as ALL,

but they are similar in many ways.

Whenever we use the words "acute leukemia,"

we are talking about AML as well as ALL.

normal
granulocyte

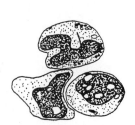

myeloblasts

★ How Doctors Know You Have Leukemia

Your body is a wonderful thing

but it is not perfect.

Sometimes something goes wrong.

It can be hurt on the outside.

You might fall down and skin your knee.

When something goes wrong on the outside of you,

you know a lot about it.

You can see it and touch it.

Your doctor can see it and touch it, too.

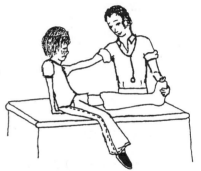

Just by looking, your doctor will know

if you are getting better.

Something can go wrong on your inside, too.

You can't see it or touch it,

but it's wrong just the same.

Only it's harder to understand.

It's harder for your doctor, too.

But doctors have special ways

to see what's going on inside you.

Many of these ways are used to find out

if you have leukemia.

Every disease has symptoms.

Symptoms are the things you feel or notice

that aren't right.

Symptoms are the reasons that you go to the doctor.

The doctor will ask you questions about your symptoms.

This is called "taking a history."

That is how the doctor gets the first clues

about what disease you have.

What were your symptoms?

What do you think other symptoms might be?

The most common symptoms of acute leukemia are:

1. feeling tired all the time

2. fever

3. easy bruising or bleeding

4. bone pain

5. large lymph nodes

6. big swollen tummy

7. getting a lot of infections

8. funny bumps on your body or head

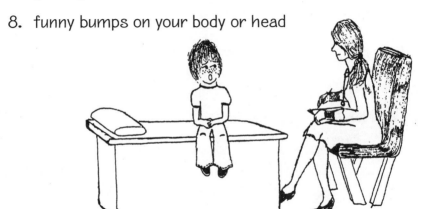

Every disease has signs.

Signs are what the <u>doctor</u> finds

when he or she is examining you.

They tell your doctor that something isn't right.

Do you remember what your signs were?

What do you think other signs might be?

The most common signs of acute leukemia are:

1. pale skin and gums
2. fever
3. bruises and petechiae (page 28)
4. tender bones
5. big lymph nodes
6. big spleen and liver
7. funny bumps on your body or head

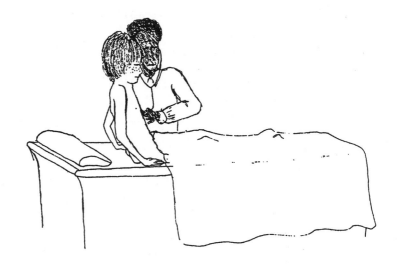

Probably when you went to your doctor,

you had some of these symptoms and signs.

You may have had them for only a few days.

You may have had them for a few months.

These symptoms and signs happen with other diseases, too.

So if you had only one or two at the beginning,

your doctor might not have thought of leukemia right away.

Most children have fevers at one time or another.

Most children have bruises and aches at one time or another.

Most children have big lymph nodes at one time or another.

That makes it difficult to know exactly what's wrong, at first.

So, sometimes, doctors and parents wait to see

what else will happen.

If it's not leukemia, it will go away.

And usually it's <u>not</u> leukemia.

If it's a different disease, time will tell.

And usually it <u>is</u> a different disease.

If it is leukemia, more symptoms and signs will show up.

Then, if the doctor thinks that you might have leukemia

or another blood disease,

you will have to get your blood looked at.

◇Blood Tests

For doctors to look at your blood,

they have to get a little bit of it from you.

This is done in one of two ways.

The easiest way is just to make a little prick

in one of your fingers.

Another way is to put a needle into one of your veins.

If you have leukemia

you already know how blood tests are done—

but what happens to the blood when the doctors have it?

If the doctor thinks you have leukemia,

he or she will want to look at your blood carefully.

A drop of your blood will be put on a glass slide

and spread out until it's very thin.

Then the doctor will look at it through a microscope—

a special instrument that makes tiny things

like blood cells

look very big indeed.

glass slide

The doctor wants to know if all the cells

that should be there, are there.

Do all the cells look like they are supposed to?

And most important, are there any blasts?

Often, just by looking at the blood,

doctors can learn what kind of disease you have.

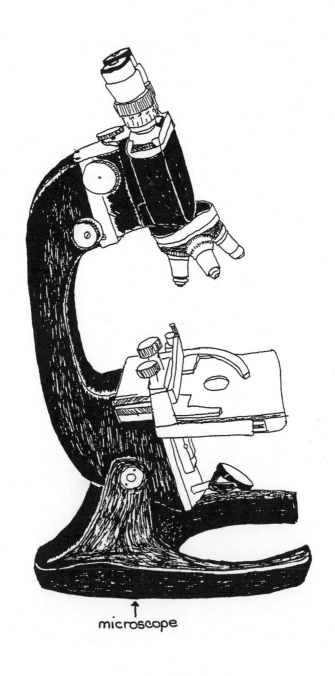

microscope

All your different kinds of cells

will be counted, too, by a person or a machine.

By counting the number of cells

in the same certain tiny amount of blood

from many people for many years,

doctors have figured out how many of each cell

should be in that amount.

These "how many's" are called "normal values."

Normal values are helpful,

but since no two people are exactly the same,

it doesn't necessarily mean someone is sick

if their counts are not the same as the normal values.

Most people have counts that are normal.

Some healthy people never do.

Some have normal counts for years

and then suddenly change, for no obvious reason.

It is the change that makes doctors worry.

If your counts change from what is normal for you

to something else—whether to a higher or a lower value—

your doctors will want to know why.

Your counts will probably come back to your doctor or nurse

on a computer screen.

You can ask to have a copy printed out for you

so you and your family can keep up with your counts.

The complete blood count (CBC) looks at the big picture.

The important numbers to look at on your CBC are listed here.

"WBC" is how many white cells you have.

Normal is about 4,000 to 11,000.

"RBC" is how many red cells you have.

Normal is about 5.00 to 6.00.

"HGB" (hemoglobin) and "HCT" (hematocrit) tell you

how well your red cells are doing the job of carrying oxygen.

HGB is normally between 11 and 14 for children.

HCT is usually between 36.0 and 48.0.

"Platelets" tells you how many platelets you have.

Normal is between about 130,000 and 400,000.

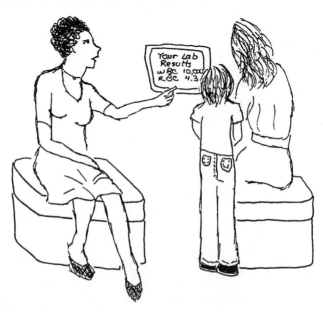

Another kind of count is the differential count, or "diff."

You can also get a printout of this count.

What are all those things on the diff?

To begin with, the diff will show the CBC counts

you already know about.

But it has extra added attractions,

especially more information about your white cells.

You already know that there are three main kinds:

granulocytes, lymphocytes and monocytes.

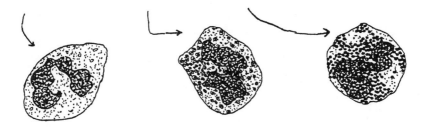

You don't know, though, that there are also

three different kinds of normal granulocytes:

neutrophils, eosinophils and basophils.

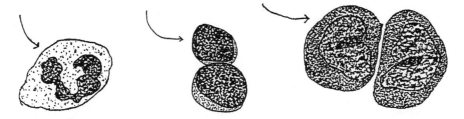

"Seg" and "band" are just descriptions of

two different ways that neutrophils can look.

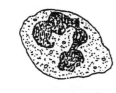

" seg " neutrophil

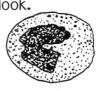

" band" neutrophil

69

"Atypical lymphocytes" just means funny-looking lymphocytes.

In some diseases caused by viruses

the lymphocytes don't look normal at all.

But when the disease goes away, they look normal again.

Many of the other words are names for cells

normally found in bone marrow—but not in blood.

These are immature cells, but they are not leukemic blasts.

Progranulocytes, myelocytes and metamyelocytes

are immature granulocytes.

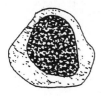
progranulocyte

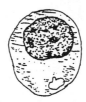
myelocyte

metamyelocyte

Prolymphocytes are immature lymphocytes.

Promonocytes are immature monocytes.

You already know what blasts are.

They mean leukemia.

But the immature forms do not always mean leukemia.

Other diseases and sometimes medicines

can cause these cells to appear.

Now that the doctors know you have leukemia,

they will want to look at your blood often. Why?

1. to see if there are any blasts in your blood
2. to make sure that the medicines you will be taking to

   kill your leukemia cells

   don't hurt your normal cells too much

So blood tests are going to be regular things for you.

Some time, why don't you ask your doctor

if you can look at your own blood through the microscope?

You can get copies of your counts,

only don't worry if they are lower than normal.

Many of the medicines you will get

will make your counts lower than usual,

especially your WBC and platelet counts.

Low counts will be normal for you.

Your doctors will try to make sure that your counts

don't get low enough to cause you trouble.

If your counts get too low

your doctors may change the amounts of the medicines you take

until your counts get back up to where they should be.

When you have leukemia,

blood tests are an important part of your life.

◇Bone Marrow Aspirations

There is one more test that your doctor used

to know for sure that you have leukemia.

This is the bone marrow test.

Sometimes blasts don't show up in the blood

even when the bone marrow is full of them.

So the doctors looked at your bone marrow

to be sure that you have leukemia.

You have probably already had your first "bone marrow."

You will have to have more bone marrows

in the weeks, months and years to come.

You won't have as many bone marrows as blood tests,

but every now and again doctors will want to check it

for the same reasons they want to check your blood:

1. to see if there are blasts in your marrow
2. to make sure that the medicines you will be taking

    to kill your leukemia cells

    don't hurt your normal cells too much

Many people with leukemia, grownups as well as kids,

think the bone marrow test

is the worst thing about having leukemia.

For one thing, it just plain hurts

to have some bone marrow taken out of you.

Luckily, there are lots of ways to make the test hurt less

or not at all.

One way is to use your imagination.

While the test is being done,

you can just pretend you are somewhere else,

someplace you really like to be,

doing something you really like to do.

It's only pretend, of course, but pretending can be powerful—

so powerful that it can make bone marrow tests less painful.

The trick to the imagination way

is to stay in your special place no matter what—

and to remember to keep

breathing slowly in and out

no matter what.

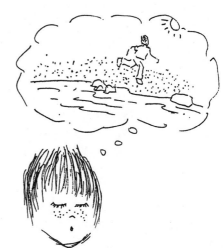

The imagination way doesn't work for everyone,

so doctors have other things they can do to help you.

One is a magic medicine called EMLA.

It looks just like toothpaste.

magic EMLA !

A small amount of the EMLA cream is put on the place

where the bone marrow test will be done

about an hour or two ahead of time.

The EMLA is kept in place by a sticky, see-through little sheet

that kind of looks like Saran Wrap.

This lets you keep your clothes on

while you wait for the EMLA to work.

Ask your nurse if you can put some EMLA on your hand

so you can see what it looks and feels like.

EMLA (and other medicines like it) is great stuff.

It makes your skin's pain nerves go completely asleep

and stay that way through the whole test,

so you won't feel anything when the needle goes in.

You're awake, but your skin's pain nerves aren't.

You may feel other funny feelings, but you won't hurt.

EMLA is an example of a kind of anesthesia

(anesthesia means "no pain")

that can be used to make lots of tests less painful—

not just bone marrows.

EMLA inside

Another idea is to make <u>you</u> so sleepy
you don't care what is going on.
This is done by giving you a medicine, like Versed,
shortly before the bone marrow test.
Yet another way is to use a medicine
to put you completely asleep.
This way is called "general anesthesia,"
because it affects your whole body,
not just one part like EMLA does.

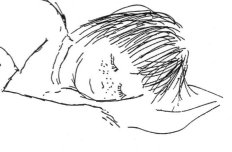

General anesthesia really works, but it is more complicated
for you and for everyone taking care of you.
For one thing, you usually can't eat or drink anything
except maybe some clear liquids like water
from the night before general anesthesia is going to be used
until after the test is done and you are completely awake.

You and your parents and your doctor
need to discuss all the ways there are to help you not hurt
during bone marrow tests
—or any other tests or procedures you may have—
to decide what is best for you.
One thing is for sure:

    👀 <u>You do not have to feel pain during tests and
procedures anymore.</u>

Another reason many people don't like bone marrow tests

is that they are done on your back—

and you can't see what's happening.

There is a lot you can do about that.

The next few pages will show you what happens.

You can also ask your doctor or nurse

to show you the bone marrow room.

You can see all the stuff they use to do the test.

You can do a pretend bone marrow yourself

on a doll or stuffed animal,

with your doctor or nurse helping you.

Some treatment centers also have videotapes

showing bone marrow tests and other procedures

that you and your parents can watch.

All of these ways of seeing how bone marrows

are done on others

can help you "see" what is happening to you.

Then it's not so mysterious or scary.

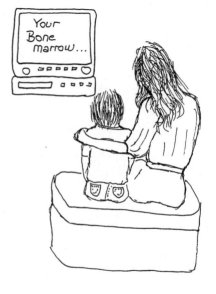

To look at your bone marrow,

doctors must get a sample of it.

Bone marrow is inside your bones,

so it's harder to get than blood is.

Doctors will usually take marrow out

through a needle

from the back of your hip bones,

but they could use your breast bone,

the front of your hip bone

or even one of your back bones.

Sometimes they use

the shin bone in tiny babies.

The reason they use these bones

is that they are close to your skin

and contain the most marrow cells,

which makes it a lot easier on you,

besides being easier for the doctor.

Bone marrow can be taken out of your

bones three ways:

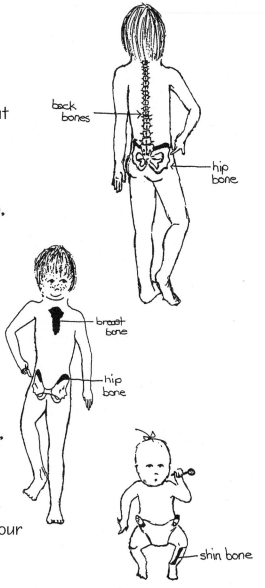

1. aspiration (which is like sucking some out through a thin straw)

2. biopsy (which is taking a small piece of it)

3. trephine (which is taking a tiny piece of whole bone)

Often all three ways are done during a single procedure.

When you go for your bone marrow aspiration,

you will be asked to lie down on your tummy on a table.

Your pants and underpants will be pulled down a little

so that the doctor can examine your back.

Then the doctor will put on thin rubber gloves

and wipe your hip

with cold stuff that kills germs (an antiseptic).

Then he or she will put clean paper towels on you,

leaving only a little bit of your skin showing.

All of these things are done to protect you.

There are germs on your skin and on the doctor's skin, too.

No one wants those germs to get inside of you.

Gloves, towels and antiseptics keep germs away.

The needles that will be used are sterilized,

which means they don't have any germs on them.

Nothing will touch you that isn't clean.

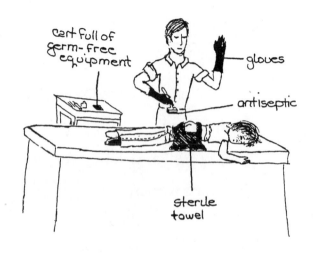

Now that you are prepared ("prepped"),

the doctor will give your back

a shot of numbing medicine (Xylocaine).

This shot can sting if you haven't used EMLA,

or you may feel pressure or coldness if you have used EMLA.

The Xylocaine will be put where

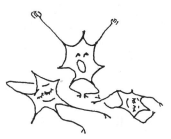

sleepy nerves

the aspiration needle will go,

all the way down to the bone.

The medicine can't be put <u>into</u> the bone,

but since bones don't have any nerves,

you don't feel pain when the needle goes into your bones.

It's just the stuff around bones that has nerves.

EMLA and Xylocaine make these nerves sleepy,

so they forget to send pain messages to your brain.

When the medication is all in,

the doctor may wait for a little while

to be sure your nerves are sound asleep.

It usually works pretty fast.

The doctor may examine your back again while waiting.

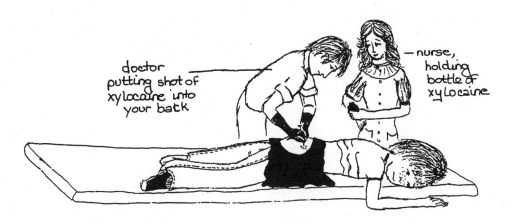

doctor putting shot of xylocaine into your back

— nurse, holding bottle of xylocaine

The doctor might then use a small scalpel

to make a tiny opening in your skin.

Then the doctor will take a special needle

and slide it past the sleepy nerves, muscle, fat and bone

right into your bone marrow.

The needle is actually two parts—a hollow tube

and a solid plug to make it strong enough to get into a bone.

When it is in, the doctor will pull out the plug

and leave the hollow tube in place.

Then the doctor will attach an empty suction tube (syringe)

to the opening of the needle

and pull some marrow out by pulling back on the plunger.

The sucking-out of the marrow is what hurts

if you haven't used EMLA or aren't sleepy or sleeping—

but it lasts only a few seconds.

When the doctor has enough marrow,

the needle may be taken out of your back.

Then you just have to wait a few minutes

until you stop bleeding,

get a bandage put on

and you're all done.

(By the way,

the bandage should stay on for a whole day.)

sleepy nerves

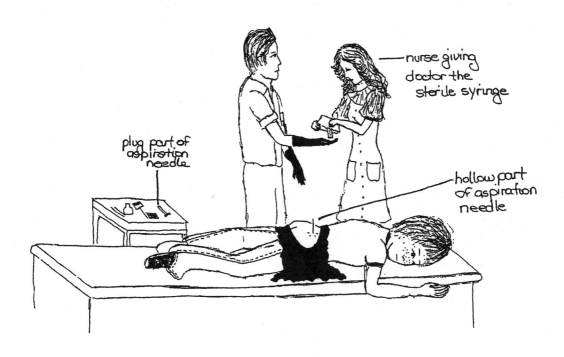

nurse giving
doctor the
sterile syringe

plug part of
aspiration
needle

hollow part
of aspiration
needle

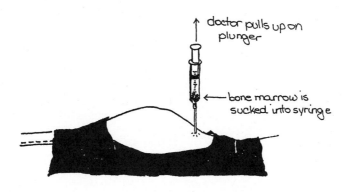

doctor pulls up on
plunger

bone marrow is
sucked into syringe

Now, sometimes the doctor won't be able to get any marrow

on the first try.

That means that a second try will have to be made.

Usually this try will work.

But sometimes, in leukemia,

the bone marrow gets packed so full of cells

that an aspiration won't work

even with two or more tries.

This is one of the times

when a biopsy can be used.

Biopsies and trephines can also be done right after

the aspiration is finished,

if your doctor thinks doing this

would help him understand better

what is happening inside your bone marrow.

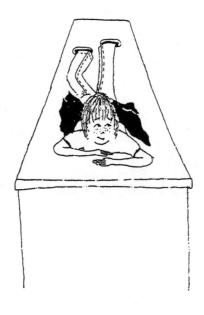

If a biopsy is going to be done,

it means that you'll have to stay still

for a few more minutes.

Then the doctor will take the hollow part of the needle

that is still in your bone

from the aspiration part

and gently push it in further

until he thinks that there is a piece of whole marrow in it.

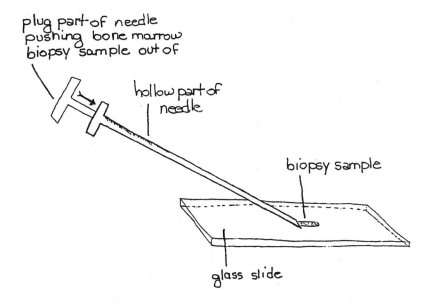

plug part of needle
pushing bone marrow
biopsy sample out of

hollow part of
needle

biopsy sample

glass slide

Then the needle will be taken out

and the doctor will make sure

the biopsy sample is a good one.

If it is, you're all done

except for your bandage.

If it's not, the doctor may want to try again.

It would be nice if doctors could always

get a good biopsy sample

the very first time.

But sometimes it's just not possible.

If the doctor has to try again,

don't worry.

Your back is—or you are—still asleep or sleepy.

And the biopsy won't take long.

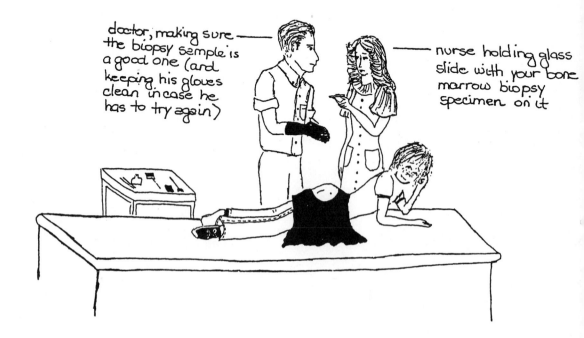

doctor, making sure the biopsy sample is a good one (and keeping his gloves clean in case he has to try again)

nurse holding glass slide with your bone marrow biopsy specimen on it

What the doctors do with your bone marrow

is pretty much the same as what they do

with your blood.

They study it through a microscope

and see how it looks.

They will count all the cells.

They will look for blasts.

Then they will know just how you are doing.

Why don't you ask your doctor to let you

look at your own bone marrow

through a microscope?

It's even prettier than blood

because it has more different kinds of cells.

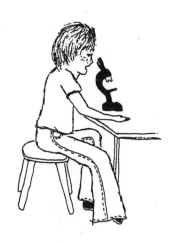

★How Doctors Treat Leukemia

Now that you know you have leukemia,

what can be done to make you better?

Fifty years ago, there was nothing that could be done.

But since then, doctors and scientists have found medicines

that kill leukemia cells.

They found each of these medicines by trying them out

on animals with leukemia,

and then on people with leukemia.

Later, doctors found out that

using many medicines at one time (combination chemotherapy)

worked better than using one medicine alone.

The treatment that you will get

will be based on the best one that's been found so far.

But new trials with new medicines

or new combinations of medicines,

as well as doses of medicines and schedules

of when to use which medicine,

are still going on to make

treatment even better.

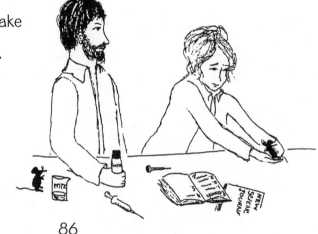

You may be asked to be part of

an experimental treatment program called a "clinical trial."

In a clinical trial, you may be asked

to try some of these new medicines,

or "investigational drugs."

Clinical trials are designed by scientists and doctors

from all over the world, who work together in large groups

such as the Children's Oncology Group (COG).

Clinical trials are very complicated programs.

They are usually written out in booklets called "protocols."

If you are "on study" or "on a protocol,"

you will get exactly the same treatment all the children

in that study will get—no matter where you or they live.

If you decide to be in a clinical trial

and it is comparing different treatments,

you will get the best of the proven medicines

or the best of the new investigational drugs.

If you decide not to be part of a clinical trial,

you can still have the best of the proven medicines.

Not all people decide to be part of a clinical trial.

Most people do, though.

You and your family have to decide for you.

Not all people are asked to be part of a clinical trial.

Your doctor will consider everything about you and your leukemia

in deciding exactly what the best way is to treat your leukemia.

Before we go any further on treatment,

a few things need to be said.

You and your parents—

and maybe your pets or dolls or stuffed animals—

are the experts on you.

Your doctors and nurses are the experts on leukemia.

Most doctors agree

that leukemia is a tricky disease to treat.

Your regular doctor will probably want you

to have your leukemia treated at a place

where the doctors and nurses

are really good at treating leukemia.

There are a lot of treatment centers like this.

Your doctor may already work at one of them.

If not, then your doctor will tell your family to take you to one.

That's not because your regular doctor

doesn't like you anymore.

It's because your doctor wants you to get the very best care.

Your regular doctor will still be

there for you for all the ordinary

stuff that comes up

while you have leukemia

and after.

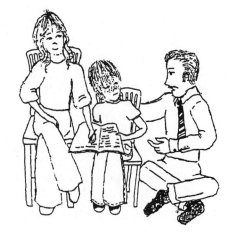

Choosing a treatment center, though, can be confusing.

Everyone you and your parents know,

not just your doctor,

will have ideas about this.

Even people you <u>don't</u> know will have ideas,

if you use a computer to go on the Internet.

If you trust your doctor, let your doctor guide you.

Your doctor knows you and likes you.

If you find you don't like your doctor's choice,

you can go to another center and get a second opinion.

You can see what the other center looks like and feels like.

But don't spend too much time running around

trying to find the perfect place.

Any center that is involved

in a major clinical trials group

like the one mentioned on page 87

will be able to give you treatment

that is the best there is on earth

right now.

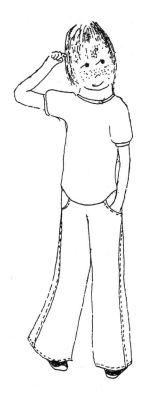

The main idea in treating your leukemia

is to get you into a state called remission.

Remission is not a state like California or Texas or Iowa.

Remission is when you don't have any

symptoms or signs of leukemia,

and when your blood and bone marrow tests

don't show any leukemia cells.

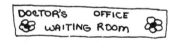 <u>Remission is not the same as being cured.</u>

Many people are staying in remission for so many years

that they are considered to be cured.

They have grown up, gotten married, had families and jobs.

Most important, they are healthy.

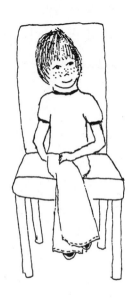

But for now, getting you into remission

and keeping you there is the main goal.

Once you are in remission,

you can live a pretty normal life.

You'll just have to go to the doctor

more often than most people

for a while.

The way doctors get you into remission
is by a process called "induction."
During induction, doctors use many medicines
to try to kill every leukemia cell in your body.
Induction usually takes about a month.
The medicines you will be given will be chosen
especially for you, based on things like
how old you are, how much you weigh,
what kind of leukemia you have and if you are in a clinical trial.
If you have ALL, most of your treatment, including induction,
will be done in a clinic or day hospital
and you usually won't have to stay there overnight.
If you have AML, most of your treatment will be done in a
hospital, and you often will have to stay there for a while.
You need to be in these special places
because the medicines used to kill leukemia cells
are extremely strong.
Your doctors want to be sure your body can handle them.
Also, many of the medicines used in the early part of treatment
have to be put directly into one of your veins (intravenous, or IV).
(There is a whole section on treatment later in this book.
It describes all the medicines and procedures you may have
as part of your treatment—including a way
to make the IVs and blood tests less of a problem—
during induction and after.)

This page is for you,

your parents and your doctor to use

to write down your induction program.

❋ MY INDUCTION PROGRAM ❋

What happens next depends on what kind of leukemia you have.

If you have ALL, for the next month or so

you will get some new medicines

that will attack any leftover blasts.

This is called "consolidation."

While induction is kind of like learning

how to throw, catch and bat,

consolidation is like playing

an actual T-ball, baseball or softball game.

The rest of this page is for you

to write down your consolidation program.

❃ MY CONSOLIDATION PROGRAM ❃

The next part of your ALL treatment is called

"interim maintenance."

"Interim" means "in between."

"Maintenance" means keeping things the way they are.

With leukemia, maintenance means using medicines

to make sure your leukemia doesn't come back.

The two months of interim maintenance

is kind of a recovery time for your body,

but a lot is still going on.

It's sort of like the practices

a winning T-ball, baseball or softball team has

between the time it wins its last regular game

and the time it plays in the league championship game.

The rest of this page is for you

to write down your interim maintenance program.

❈ MY INTERIM MAINTENANCE PROGRAM ❈

The championship game in the treatment of ALL

is called "delayed intensification."

"Delayed" means "after a while."

"Intensification" is something like really trying hard

to do one thing perfectly.

The delayed intensification part of treating ALL

is the final big attack on any leukemia cells

that may still be hiding in your body.

(Both delayed intensification and interim maintenance

may be done more than once.)

If you have AML, after induction

you skip straight to this part of treatment.

Only because there aren't other steps in between,

for AML this phase is simply called "intensification."

You go to the championship game right away.

❈ MY DELAYED INTENSIFICATION PROGRAM ❈

or

❈ MY INTENSIFICATION PROGRAM ❈

Once you are finished with the intensification part of your

treatment and are well into a good remission

(most people get into a good remission),

the next step is called maintenance therapy.

You already know what maintenance means:

keeping things the way they are.

Whether you have ALL or AML,

you will be given yet another combination of medicines

to maintain your remission.

If you have ALL,

you will stay on maintenance therapy for about 1½ to 3½ years

depending on whether you are a girl or a boy

and on when interim maintenance started.

(Keeping boys with ALL in remission

takes some extra time—no one knows why.)

The exact medicines you take

during your maintenance may change

depending on what is found to work best for you.

The good part is,

you don't have to go to the clinic nearly as often.

In fact, your life will start feeling pretty normal again.

The next page is for you, your parents

and your doctor to use

to write down your maintenance program.

❀ MY MAINTENANCE PROGRAM ❀

If you have AML,

another form of treatment may be considered

once you have completed consolidation therapy.

It is called a bone marrow transplant.

How it is done is described later in this book.

In a bone marrow transplant,

all of your bone marrow is killed

and replaced with healthy bone marrow

from someone who doesn't have leukemia.

Sounds simple, doesn't it?

It's not.

A bone marrow transplant is probably the most

intensive kind of treatment of all,

so it isn't done unless your leukemia

is more likely to cause you serious problems

than the bone marrow transplant is.

AML blasts are harder to kill with medicines than ALL blasts,

so super-intensive treatment during the first remission

makes sense in AML.

But not for ALL,

because the first remission can last . . . forever.

Bone marrow transplant is reserved for all people with AML,

all adults with ALL,

all children with chronic (instead of acute) leukemias

and those children with ALL who don't get better

with medicines alone.

The reason bone marrow transplants are done at all

is because of a big problem with leukemia.

Remissions don't always last long enough.

Sometimes leukemia comes back

(this is called a "relapse").

When a relapse happens,

it's like starting all over again.

Your doctors will try to get you into another remission.

With ALL, doctors are usually successful

in getting a second remission.

But if there are other relapses after that,

it gets harder and harder to get you into remission again.

With AML, adult ALL and chronic leukemia in children,

it is extremely hard for doctors to get

even a second remission.

So everyone tries to make each remission last

as long as possible.

And if the right generous healthy person is found

who can share bone marrow with you,

this is when and why a bone marrow transplant will be tried.

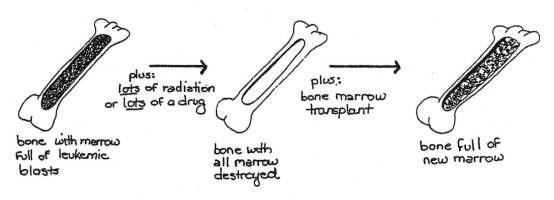

plus:
lots of radiation
or lots of a drug

plus:
bone marrow
transplant

bone with marrow
full of leukemic
blasts

bone with
all marrow
destroyed

bone full of
new marrow

Maybe you won't go into remission.

The treatment is good and usually works, but it's not perfect.

That is why enjoying every healthy day is very important.

If your leukemia gets out of control, it can take your life.

If your doctors aren't able to get you into remission—

whether it's the first time they try or after a relapse—

they want you to know this: all that is possible to do to keep

you comfortable and free from pain will be done for you,

whether you and your family decide you should

spend this time in the hospital or at home.

If you decide to be in the hospital,

your parents can stay with you there.

Your friends from the clinic can visit.

Your doctors and nurses will be there.

You won't be alone.

If you decide you want to be at home,

your family should ask your doctor

about something called hospice.

Hospice doctors, nurses and health aides

can help make this a better time for you and your family.

Only you and your family can decide what is right for you.

But even at this time, you all have the power

to make important decisions

about your life.

This is the last page of the general section about treatment.

It is a good place to talk about forms of treatment

that you might hear about

from friends, neighbors or relatives,

or at the health food store or on the Internet.

There are many things that are claimed

to cure all forms of cancer.

They include vitamins, special diets, herbs

and certain "medicines."

Some faith healers say they can cure cancer.

The medical profession in the United States

does not think that these so-called cures work.

However, some people think that they have nothing to lose

by trying one or another of these methods.

No one can tell you what to do.

If you want to try one of these "cures,"

all we can do is ask

that you discuss it with your doctors first.

You have a lot to gain from regular care.

> ∞ Most important, never take any medicine of any kind—
> even a "natural" herbal medicine—
> unless your doctor says it's OK.

It could keep your leukemia medicines

from doing their job.

★Complications of Leukemia

You know how important it is

that all of your cells and organs and systems

work right and work together.

So it's easy to figure out that when

something goes wrong with one part of you,

all of you is affected.

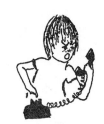

In a city, if the telephone lines fall down,

everybody is affected.

If you have ALL, only your lymphocytes are malignant.

If you have AML, only your granulocytes are malignant.

But all of your body is affected.

The other things that can go wrong

are called complications.

If any of these complications happen to you,

doctors will try to treat them, too.

Only a part of the treatment of leukemia

is aimed at killing leukemia cells—

the rest is aimed at taking care of you.

There are seven common complications of leukemia:

1. Anemia (see pages 26-27)

If your red blood cell count gets too low,

you may need to have a blood transfusion.

This is when you are given blood from a healthy person.

It will give you the red cells you need to carry oxygen.

More about blood transfusions

can be found on pages 177 to 187.

2. Thrombocytopenia (see pages 28-29)

If you don't have enough platelets,

your blood vessels may begin to leak.

How serious this complication is

depends on where the leaky blood vessels are.

If they're in your arms or legs, you'll get a bruise

or maybe a big lump of blood called a hematoma.

Because this lump can push against nearby nerves,

it can be painful.

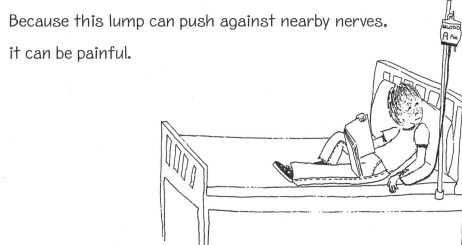

The most serious place for leaky blood vessels to be
is inside your head.
The reason is that your brain
can't move out of the way of the blood or hematoma
(a glob of blood)
the way the muscles in your leg can.
That's because your brain is surrounded by bone
and bone doesn't stretch like skin does.
If the vessel is leaking slowly,
you might get a headache that won't go away
or things might start looking all blurry.
If the vessel is leaking quickly,
you may suddenly be unable to move or talk
or even become unconscious (sort of like fainting).
Your family and friends should know
that if something like this happens
to call your doctor right away
and take you to a hospital.

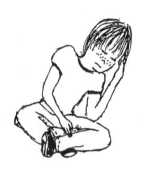

Bleeding is a common complication

in all types of leukemia.

When you are in remission,

it won't be much of a problem.

Lots of people in remission

play football and other sports without danger.

If you fall down hard and get a bruise,

you probably would have gotten it even without leukemia.

But if you get bruises without bumping yourself,

your doctor should know.

If your platelet count gets too low,

you may need to have a platelet transfusion.

In fact, a platelet transfusion may be

one of the first things that happens to you

once your leukemia is diagnosed.

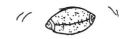

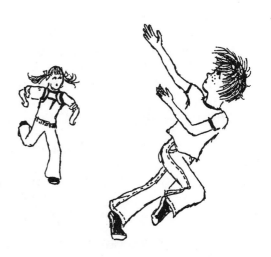

3. Infections (see pages 30-34)

Infections can happen when your white count gets too low,

or just because your WBCs aren't working too well.

If you get a bacterial infection, you will be given medicines

called antibiotics to help your body fight the infection.

For most of the time you are in treatment, and for a while after,

you'll probably be taking an antibiotic called Bactrim.

Bactrim prevents a common kind of lung infection,

called Pneumocystis, that people whose immune systems

aren't working well can get.

If you get a serious infection,

you may have to be in the hospital for a while.

You can do a lot to prevent infections.

You can take good care of yourself by taking baths,

by washing your hands often, by getting enough sleep and food.

You can take good care of your teeth

by doing exactly what your dentist tells you to do.

You can stay away from people who have infections.

This doesn't mean that you shouldn't go to school

or play outside or spend time with people you like.

Having fun is an important part of living and staying healthy.

It's just that if you know someone has a disease

that you might catch—why take chances?

If you are accidentally exposed to a viral disease,

especially chicken pox or regular measles, tell your doctor.

If you do get sick, tell someone.

It may just be a dumb old cold

for which there is no real treatment.

But if it seems to be more than that, go see your doctor—

just as you would if you didn't have leukemia.

If you are feeling sick for no reason

or you suddenly get a high fever

or you get all hot and sweaty one minute

and cold and shivery the next,

you may have an infection.

Sometimes it's not easy for the doctor

to figure out where in your body

the infection is located

or what kind of germ is causing it.

The doctor has to know these things

to give you the right treatment.

You can help by telling the doctor

as much as you can about how you feel

and how you think you got the infection.

When the doctor examines you,

she will get more clues.

X-rays, especially of the chest and bones,

are also very helpful.

(They are also fun to look at.)

The best way to know what germ is causing your infection

is to try to get some of the germs

and grow them outside your body.

This is called "culturing."

Depending on where your doctor thinks

your infection is located,

she or he may want to culture samples

of your urine, blood or spinal fluid (see pages 163-168).

If your doctor thinks you have pneumonia,

he may want to have a small piece of your lung (a biopsy)

both to culture and to look at under a microscope.

Cultures and biopsies are important

when you have an infection.

Medicines that work well against one germ

often don't work well against others.

So cultures and biopsies tell your doctor

not only what germ is causing your infection

but also what medicine can cure it.

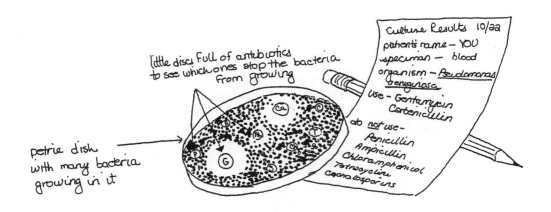

little discs full of antibiotics to see which ones stop the bacteria from growing

petrie dish with many bacteria growing in it

Culture Results 10/22
patient's name — YOU
specimen — blood
organism — Pseudomonas
   aeruginosa
use — Gentamycin
   Carbenicillin
do not use —
   Penicillin
   Ampicillin
   Chloramphenicol
   Tetracycline
   Cephalosporins

4. CNS leukemia

You already know that leukemia cells—blasts—

can be in other places besides bone marrow.

One place where blasts like to hide

is in the central nervous system (CNS).

This is your brain and your spinal cord

and the envelope around them, called the meninges.

All around your brain and spinal cord,

inside the meninges,

is a clear liquid called cerebrospinal fluid,

or CSF for short.

Sometimes blasts sneak into the CSF and hide there

and don't cause any symptoms at all, at first.

After a while, though, they can cause trouble.

This trouble is called CNS leukemia

(or meningeal leukemia).

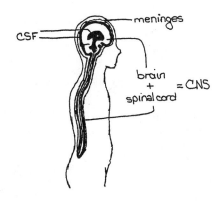

The symptoms of CNS leukemia are:

1. bad headaches that don't go away
2. vomiting for no reason
3. weight gain while off prednisone
   (a medicine used to treat leukemia)
4. blurry or double vision

Some of these symptoms can happen with other diseases,
such as flu.
But if the symptoms don't go away,
please call your doctor.
The most common sign of CNS leukemia
is called papilledema.
The doctor finds it by looking into your eyes.
Papilledema is a special way
the inside of your eye looks
when there's too much pressure behind it.
In CNS leukemia, the pressure of the CSF is high.
That is why your doctor will look into your eyes
every time you visit the clinic.

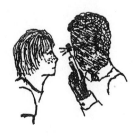

You may have already had medication by spinal tap
(see pages 163-168).
and maybe radiation therapy (see pages 169-176).
to try to prevent CNS leukemia from happening.
Unfortunately, medication and radiation therapy
don't always work.
If you <u>get</u> CNS leukemia,
you will probably have to have another series of spinal taps
and radiation therapy, if you haven't already had it
or if you haven't had all the radiation
that is safe for you.
This is the only way there is to treat it at this time,
but we are always trying to find new ways.

5. Bone pain

Leukemia can make the bone marrow so crowded
that it pushes on the hard part of the bone
and causes it to hurt.
If your bones ache a lot
or if you get a hard bump on a bone
tell your doctor.
The pain usually goes away
soon after treatment is started.

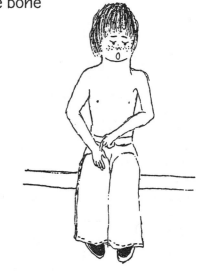

6. Kidney problems (see page 15)

When cells are dividing often (in leukemia)

or when they are dying in large numbers (in treatment),

they make lots of a substance called uric acid.

Uric acid can plug up your kidneys,

so it is harder for your body to get rid of wastes.

Luckily, this complication usually only happens during the first

days of treatment, and it's usually easy to take care of.

Your job is to drink lots of liquids

to help your kidneys not get plugged up.

A chemical called "bicarb" can be added to your IV line.

This chemical helps the body not have problems with uric acid.

There is also a pill called allopurinol

that stops uric acid from forming.

Most of the time, you will only have to take allopurinol

when you are first starting your treatments.

Or you may never need to take it.

If the problem is bad,

the doctors may have to delay other forms of treatment

until they're sure that your kidneys are OK.

If your kidneys stop working completely

(this almost never happens),

you can be connected to a machine

that thinks it's a kidney and it will take over

until your kidneys can do their own work again.

It's almost never that serious, so don't worry.

7. Testicular leukemia (see page 14)

A boy's private parts are called "testes."

If you are a boy, your testes are found

in the sack (scrotum) between your legs.

Sometimes leukemia blasts like to go and grow

in your testes.

This is called testicular leukemia.

It doesn't happen often,

but it can happen while you're still in bone marrow remission.

If leukemia cells go and grow in your testes,

your testes can get very swollen.

It may not hurt, but it can be frightening.

If your doctor thinks your testes

have leukemic blasts growing in them,

he or she may want to do a biopsy

(take a tiny piece of one of your testes

to look at under a microscope).

If your doctor finds blasts,

you may need to have radiation therapy to your testes

or a change in your medicines.

This section on complications
is not meant to worry you.
But it's good to be aware
of problems that may come up.
You will know—and your parents will know—
when something isn't right with you.
Some people call it "intuition."
You know best.
When you think something is wrong,
please call your doctor.

And you know what?
Your doctors like to know about
all of the things that go right, too.

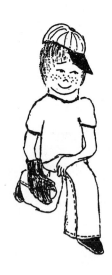

A Day
at a Time

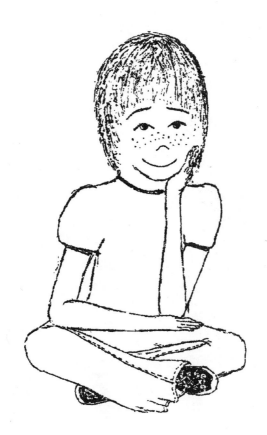

★Living with Leukemia

You will create most of this chapter for yourself

by living your own life, a day at a time.

Everyone who worked on this book

hopes that your life will be long and fun and happy.

We hope that you'll feel good most of the time.

We have some suggestions that may help you.

Your life won't be like everyone else's,

but then, no two lives are ever the same.

Leukemia will change your life.

Not only that, it will affect

the way your family lives.

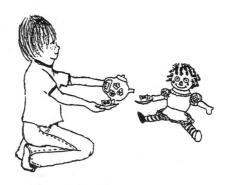

One thing you or your parents may want to do

is use a date book or calendar to keep records.

If you have a computer, that's another good way.

You can use these tools to keep track of medicines

you are supposed to take on certain days

(be sure to record when you have taken them).

You can keep track of clinic visits, too.

That way babysitters can be lined up way in advance

if you have brothers and sisters who need someone at home.

You can also keep a list of questions

you and your parents want to ask your doctor,

or a list of things you want to tell your doctor,

in a special folder.

You can also keep copies of your blood counts in the folder.

If you go away on vacation, you can take this folder with you

just in case something comes up.

If you take your calendar and folder with you to the clinic,

you'll be able to mark down any changes

in your therapy or counts.

(If your calendar is on a laptop or hand-held computer,

you can use it to play games, too!)

When you go to the clinic or the office or the hospital,
you'll have lots of friends besides your doctors.
They are all there to help you,
each in his or her own way.
You can use the next blank pages to draw pictures
of your clinic friends.
Or you could ask them for photographs of themselves
and glue the photographs to these pages.
All of these different people are interested in you—
not just in your leukemia.

Nurses, like doctors, do many different things.
Usually they will give your medicines to you.
Sometimes they do special procedures, too,
like bone marrow tests or spinal taps.
They have lots of practical advice to give you about
things like what to do about side effects of your medicines.
They are good listeners and good friends,
and often they are specialists in taking care of people
with leukemia, like you.

The receptionist arranges your appointments
and greets you at every clinic visit.
The receptionist's most important job
is to make sure the doctor has enough time
to spend with you and all the other patients.

The person who draws your blood for tests

may be a nurse or a specially trained lab technician.

The person who examines your blood under the microscope

and performs other tests on it may be a doctor

or a medical technician.

Medical technicians are experts in the laboratory,

and you don't often get to meet them, unless you try.

You'll have other special friends at the clinic or day hospital,

such as the social worker, the health educator,

the psychologist and the psychiatrist.

There are also fun friends called child life specialists.

A lot of kids call them "the playroom people,"

because they love to play with you.

Some problems just can't be fixed up with a shot or pills.

Sometimes you or your parents need to talk to someone.

These friends like to talk with people and have lots of time

just for you

if you or your parents want or need to talk.

They can help you get your thoughts together

and be better able to face—and solve—problems.

They will also come to visit you if you have to be in the hospital.

That's because they like people a lot

and know that you don't stop being a person

and having confusing problems

just because you're in the hospital.

Medical students, interns, residents and fellows

are all young doctors who are learning about leukemia

both from the older doctors and from you.

In fact, you have a job, too.

Nobody in the clinic is "just" a patient.

Everyone, including you, is a student

learning about leukemia.

And everyone, including you,

has a lot to teach others about leukemia.

❈ MY CLINIC FRIENDS ❈

✿ MY CLINIC FRIENDS ✿

When you go to your clinic visits,

you may want to bring something along

like a favorite toy, book, hobby or small video

or computer game.

A cozy blanket or pillow can be nice, too.

Sometimes you have to wait for a long time,

and waiting is easier if you have something to do.

Another thing that might be fun

is to meet other patients and their families.

They might not have the same disease as you,

but often they'll be having some of the same problems.

You can learn a lot from each other.

You might find someone from your own town or neighborhood

and then maybe your families could arrange

to share the driving.

Or perhaps you will meet someone

who will become a very special friend to you.

You won't know unless you try.

How about it?

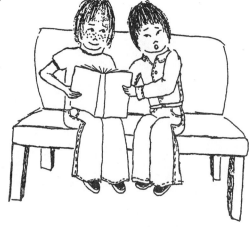

You are part of a family.

We don't know very much at all about your family,

but we do know that families get upset

when one of them has leukemia.

If you have brothers or sisters,

they may not understand what is happening to you.

They might think they somehow caused you to have leukemia

even though, of course, they didn't.

They might be afraid that they're going to get leukemia, too.

They might think your parents don't like them anymore

because they spend so much time with you.

You and your parents can do a lot to help

your brothers and sisters out.

You can tell them about leukemia

and why you have to go to the doctor so much.

You can invite them to go with you

to the clinic and show them what happens there.

You can have them meet your doctor and all your clinic friends.

You can give them this book to read.

We think that when everyone in a family understands

about leukemia and its treatment,

they won't feel left out.

Besides, if everyone knows what's going on,

you'll have lots of understanding people to talk to

if you get worried or scared.

There will be times when you <u>will</u> be

worried and scared.

Knowing you will be having a bone marrow or a spinal tap

the next time you go to the clinic

may bother you a lot.

Most people, though, get less bothered

by knowing these things in advance

than by being surprised with them

or even lied to about them.

If you don't know, you might fight the doctor

instead of helping her,

and that makes it a lot harder on both of you.

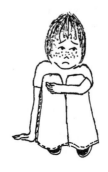

Another thing that may worry you

is having your hair fall out.

This may not ever happen to you

or it may happen more than once.

Your parents will probably worry more about this than you will,

so you might want to talk about it with them.

You will learn how they feel and they will learn how you feel.

If your hair falls out, you may want to wear a wig.

(If you think you may want a wig,

be sure to have a picture taken of you

with your hair so the wig maker

can make a wig that looks right.)

You may like a scarf or a hat better, though,

or even nothing at all.

It's OK to be bald.

Queen Elizabeth the First of England was bald.

Some movie actors and athletes are bald on purpose

because they think they look better that way.

You will have to decide how much it matters to you.

And remember—your hair almost always will grow back.

Other people may not know much about leukemia,

and they can be cruel, without meaning to be.

If other people tease you about being bald,

just tell them it's a side effect of your treatment

and that it's much more important to be healthy

than it is to have hair.

Side effects of your medications can bother you, too.

Details about these medicines can be found on pages 138 to 152.

Here are some ideas for making you feel better. . .

But first, a very important rule:

     🌀 <u>Never take any medication of any kind</u>

         <u>unless your doctor says it's OK.</u>

1. If you have an achy place in your body
   a heating pad can help, or try a hot bath.

2. If you get heartburn from prednisone or its cousin,
   dexamethasone, try eating something
   or drinking milk before you take it.
   Or you can ask your doctor
   if you can take an antacid with it.

3. If you get constipated from vincristine
   or another medicine used to treat leukemia,
   try to eat foods that contain a lot of fiber—
   fruits, vegetables, bran flakes, and whole grain breads.
   Drink a lot of apple juice or prune juice.

If constipation still bothers you, ask your doctor about it.

Your doctor may suggest that you take a laxative.

Let your doctor decide this.

4. If you gain lots of weight when you take prednisone or dexamethasone, or if your blood pressure gets too high, you should be careful not to put extra salt on your foods. Not eating salty snacks or fatty foods helps, too.

5. If you get sores in your mouth from methotrexate, you may be asked to take less of it than you usually do. You may be asked not to take it at all for a while so that your sores can heal. They will.

In the meantime, there are things you can do to help your mouth heal. Be sure to rinse out your mouth and brush your teeth after you eat. Spicy, salty foods can make your mouth feel worse— and so can lemon and other citrus juices. You might also ask your doctor if he knows of anything that could cause the nerves in your mouth to take a short nap. This would give you a rest from the discomfort.

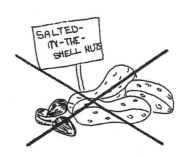

6. If you have trouble with nausea

   (feeling like you're going to throw up)

   and vomiting (actually throwing up),

   which can be caused

   by many medicines used to treat leukemia,

   your doctor can give you some medicine to help you.

These medicines, called antiemetics,

almost completely prevent nausea and vomiting

if you use them the way your doctor tells you to.

Two examples of antiemetics that work really well

are Kytril (granisetron)

and Zofran (ondansetron).

Both can be given as pills or IV.

They can be used before, during and after

you get your medicines

to prevent nausea and vomiting.

7. Almost everyone agrees

   that one of the best treatments for any problem

   is loving and being loved.

You don't need a prescription for this.

If you're not feeling very good,

why not spend some time with your favorite people

doing quiet things together—

like reading stories or watching TV?

Your problems won't disappear,

but they probably won't bother you as much.

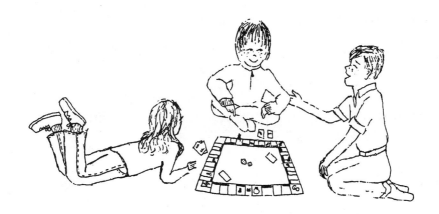

Another worry may be about school.

You'll be too busy getting your treatment

for the first 6 months or so to go to school.

Your parents need to work with your school

to help you keep up with your schoolwork.

Your treatment center may have people who can help them.

There are teachers who can come right to you

no matter where you are, at home or in the hospital.

And you can stay in touch with your classmates by phone,

e-mail and regular mail.

Your clinic friends can work with you,

your teachers and your classmates

to get everyone ready for the big day:

the day you go back to school.

On that day, you and your family

will probably be feeling a mixed-up bunch of feelings:

nervousness, excitement, happiness and fear all at once.

It's normal to feel mixed-up, strong feelings at important times.

Your going back to school means your leukemia

is under good control, maybe even gone for good.

That is a big deal.

But after a while, it will all start feeling pretty regular again.

You'll feel like you're just you and so will everyone else.

Instead of spending most of your time being a kid with leukemia,

you'll get to spend it just being a kid.

You and your family may have another big worry.

People who have leukemia don't always live as long

as other people.

What if your leukemia gets out of control?

All of us want to live a long time.

And we want the people we love to have long lives.

So these thoughts can be very upsetting to you

and the people who love you.

No one ever thinks anyone they love will get leukemia.

When it happens, some people like to pretend it isn't there.

Or they hope that it will go away if they don't talk about it.

You know better than that.

You know that you do have leukemia

and that while you probably will get better,

you may not.

If you pretend the leukemia isn't there,

you won't give yourself the very best chance

for a life that is not only long

but full of happiness, closeness and trust.

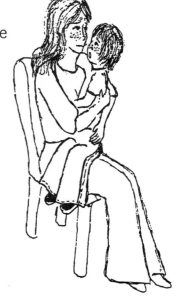

Another worry you and your family may have
will probably sound strange.
If your leukemia is cured—what then?
Will you have problems later on
because of the leukemia or its treatment?

The answer is . . . maybe.
Maybe you won't be as tall as you would have been.
Maybe you'll have problems with learning
(although you'll be just as smart as you would have been—
learning problems have nothing to do
with how smart you are).
Maybe you'll have other problems.
We'll talk more about some of these problems later.
But one thing is for sure.
If your leukemia is cured,
you will also have a lot of good things happen to you
that wouldn't happen without being cured.

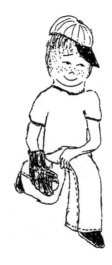

When you or a member of your family

finds that worrying is using up a lot of time and energy,

the best thing to do is to talk about your worries.

It can help to talk to your doctor, nurses,

child life specialist or social worker, too.

If you are a member of a church, synagogue or mosque

it may help you to talk to your religious leader.

It can also help a lot to join a support group

made up of other kids and families

who are also living with leukemia.

These can be real-life groups that meet

at your treatment center

or groups run by community organizations.

(There is a list of these organizations at the back of this book.)

Or, if you have a computer

you can be in a virtual support group,

one that exists in a chat room on the Internet.

(A partial list of such websites is at the back of this book.)

One thing about Internet chat rooms, though—

while the support is real and often very helpful,

the information isn't always accurate or right for you.

Always ask your doctor about anything you learn about

in a chat room

that doesn't fit with what he or she has told you.

The most important people to talk to, though,

are the people in your very own family.

Sharing your problems and worries with people you love

is another way of sharing yourself.

It doesn't mean that you are too weak

to take care of your own troubles.

It just means that you love your family so much

that you want to include them in all parts of your life.

You can keep each other from getting so worried

that no one has any fun anymore.

It's OK to be worried about having leukemia.

Everyone worries.

But try not to be afraid of living

and sharing your life with people you love.

A day at a time.

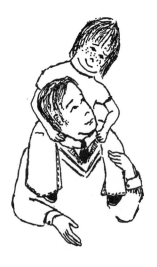

A day at a time.

Whether you have leukemia or not,

every single day is important

and always will be.

Remember that as you grow older.

Remember, too, that you are not special

because you have leukemia

or because you had it

but because you are you.

You won't stop being special if your leukemia is cured.

Your brothers and sisters are special

even though they haven't had leukemia.

When you are feeling good,

you'll still have to do your chores and homework.

You'll still lose baseball and soccer games

(because the ump or ref made a bad call, of course).

You'll have plain, old, ordinary days

with plain, old, ordinary problems.

And every one of those days is wonderful, too.

Because it is your day.

Treatment

Things you wanted to know but didn't think you'd understand

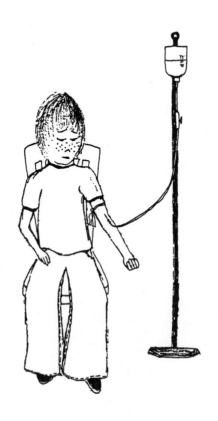

This section of the book

has more details about treatment.

Those of us who wrote this book

couldn't guess exactly what your treatment program

would be like.

So, we decided to tell about all the kinds of treatment

that are now being used.

You can read just the pages

that tell about parts of your program—

or you can read it all, if you want to.

Treating leukemia, as you will see,

is sometimes confusing and complicated.

The common methods used to kill blasts

are chemotherapy and radiation therapy.

Blood transfusions don't kill blasts,

but to some people with leukemia

they can be very important.

Bone marrow transplants and immunotherapy

are newer kinds of treatment.

They are not easy to understand,

but not impossible either.

You will hear about them,

and you may have one of them yourself.

For this reason we thought you might want to know

something about them.

★ Chemotherapy

Chemotherapy means treating a sickness

with chemicals, or medicines.

You will be given several medicines.

Each one has its own way of killing blasts.

Some only kill blasts that are dividing.

Others kill all blasts, even if they aren't dividing.

The type and amount of each medicine that you get

are figured out especially for you,

depending on how tall you are and how much you weigh.

The amounts may change as you get older and bigger.

That's why you have to be measured and weighed

every time you go to the clinic.

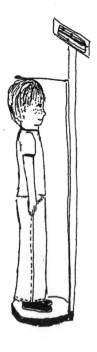

The amount of each medicine that you get

can also depend on how your body reacts to it.

Medicines that are strong enough to kill blasts

are strong enough to do other things, too.

The other things that medicines do,

besides what we want them to do, are called side effects.

Some of the side effects are unpleasant.

A few are serious.

You may have some side effects, or none at all.

It's hard to know.

But if you know about side effects and one of them happens,

you won't have to worry.

You'll know it's not your leukemia getting worse.

You and your doctors will watch for these side effects.

Some of them can be found

by doing blood tests and bone marrow aspirations.

Others can be seen when the doctor examines you.

Others you will just have to tell the doctor about.

Most side effects are not serious,

and we've already talked about some of them.

Others are more serious, and if you get those,

your doctor will want you to take

less of the medicine that is causing them—or none at all.

Stopping one medicine for a while

doesn't seem to cause your leukemia to come back,

and it makes you a lot more comfortable.

Vincristine

is also called Oncovin or VCR.

It can only be given as a shot into a vein (IV).

It comes from the periwinkle plant,

and it is one of a group of medicines called vinca alkaloids.

It acts on dividing cells and stops them from dividing.

Because not all leukemia cells are dividing at one time,

VCR is usually given once a week when you begin induction.

The hope is that each time you get VCR,

it will stop a new bunch of dividing cells.

VCR will become an old friend to you.

Side effects that VCR can cause are:

Vinca minor
the periwinkle

1. pains in arms, legs, jaw or tummy

2. tingly hands or feet

3. weakness

4. hair loss

5. burning pain and blisters where the needle went in
   if any vincristine leaked out while it was being put in

6. constipation

7. loss of appetite and mild nausea and vomiting

You will probably get only one or two of these side effects.
Maybe none at all.

Daunorubicin (daunomycin or rubidomycin or DNM)

or a closely related drug called

Adriamycin (doxorubicin or ADR)

can only be given as an IV shot.

DNM and ADR are both members

of a group of medicines called antibiotics.

They act by stopping cells from making DNA and RNA,

so that the cells can't grow and divide.

Both DNM and ADR can hurt your heart

if you get too much of them.

No one really knows how much is too much for you,

so the total amount that you get will be watched carefully.

You won't be given more than your doctors think is safe for you.

If you notice that you get short of breath—

that you can't play hard because you have trouble breathing—

please tell your doctor right away.

Other side effects that DNM or ADR can cause are:

1. nausea and vomiting
2. bone marrow depression (slowed down cell production)
3. hair loss
4. sore mouth
5. burning pain where the needle went in

You will probably get only one or two of these side effects.

Prednisone (PRED),

or a closely related medicine called dexamethasone (Decadron),

always come as pills.

If you don't know how to swallow pills,

a friend can chop them up and put them in your food.

PRED is a hormone.

It acts by killing lymphocytes.

It is usually taken for many days,

and then you may have to taper (slowly decrease) the dose

until you don't take PRED for a while.

One way of tapering is to do it by twos:

every two days, you divide the dose in half.

If your full dose is 40 mg a day,

you take only 20 mg a day (or one-half the full dose)

on the first two days of tapering.

On the next two days of tapering

you talk half of that—or 10 mg a day.

The next two days you take only 5 mg a day.

The last two days it's only 2½ mg a day.

See how easy it is?

Every two days, divide the dose in half.

You may want to use a calendar to keep track of this.

(Your doctor may want you to taper or stop PRED

using another way.)

Common side effects that PRED can cause are:

1. big appetite and weight gain,

   especially in your face and middle.

   This can happen pretty fast.

   It takes longer to go away.

   But it <u>does</u> go away when you stop taking PRED.

2. tummy aches, which could be due to a stomach ulcer,

   but usually aren't

3. not feeling ill even though you have an infection

4. mood changes (feeling either too happy or too cranky)

Other side effects that PRED can cause
(if you take it every day for a long time) are:

5. high blood sugar with thirstiness and urinating a lot

6. higher blood pressure

7. weakness

8. fragile bones

You will probably get only one or two of these side effects.
Maybe none at all.

Asparaginase

is also called Asp.

There are other forms of Asp.

One is called PEG and another Erwinia.

Asp can only be given as a shot,

usually IM (into a muscle).

It is one of a group of medicines called enzymes.

It acts by breaking up one of the ingredients

that blasts need to make protein,

and blasts need protein to grow and divide.

When you first get Asp, you may have to

be in the hospital for a few days.

Some people are very allergic to Asp.

You probably aren't, but it's best to be sure.

If you are, you will be near help.

If you aren't, you can get the rest of your Asp in the clinic.

You will have to wait in the clinic or hospital

for about an hour after you get the Asp.

This is in case you have a sudden allergic reaction,

so the doctors can give you an antiallergic medicine right away.

Because you have to wait, you might want to bring

a book to look at

or a video or computer game to play.

Side effects, besides allergy, that Asp can cause are:

1. tiredness
2. loss of appetite and weight
3. fever
4. nausea and vomiting
5. tummy ache
6. high blood sugar

   with thirstiness and frequent urinating

7. bleeding

You will probably get only one or two of these side effects. Maybe none at all.

Methotrexate

is also called amethopterin or MTX.

During induction, you may get it

as a special kind of shot into your back called a spinal tap.

This is explained later in this book.

Later on you may take it as a pill or IV or IM.

MTX is one of a group of medicines called antimetabolites.

It acts by stopping cells from making new DNA

so they can't divide.

MTX can cause two serious side effects.

One is liver damage.

Doctors can tell if this has happened by doing blood tests.

Another is lung problems, such as shortness of breath.

Again, if this happens, call your doctor.

Other side effects that MTX can cause are:

1. sores in your mouth
2. bone marrow depression
3. hair loss
4. nausea and vomiting
5. loss of appetite
6. rashes

You will probably get only one or two of these side effects.

Maybe none at all.

6-Mercaptopurine

is also called Purinethol or 6-MP.

It can be either a pill or an IV shot.

6-MP is also an antimetabolite.

6-MP can cause one serious side effect

and that is liver damage.

If that happens, you could turn yellow (jaundice).

If you get yellow, please call your doctor.

Other side effects that 6-MP can cause are:

1. bone marrow depression

2. loss of appetite

3. mild nausea and vomiting

4. sore mouth

5. diarrhea

You will probably get only one or two of these side effects.

Maybe none at all.

Cytosine arabinoside

is also called cytarabine or Cytosar or Ara-C.

It can only be given as a shot, either IV

or just under the skin (subcutaneous or SC).

It can also be given during a spinal tap.

Ara-C is another antimetabolite.

It acts by stopping cells from making DNA

so they can't divide.

Ara-C can cause one serious side effect

and that is liver damage.

Your doctors will watch for this

by doing blood tests.

Other side effects that Ara-C can cause are:

1. fever

2. loss of appetite and nausea and vomiting

3. bone marrow depression

4. stomach cramps

5. diarrhea

6. sore throat and mouth sores

7. headache

You will probably get only one or two of these side effects.

Maybe none at all.

6-Thioguanine

is also called thioguanine or 6-TG.

It comes as a pill.

It acts by stopping cells from making DNA

so they can't divide

(this is another antimetabolite).

Side effects that 6-TG can cause are:

1. bone marrow depression
2. loss of appetite
3. nausea and vomiting
4. sore mouth
5. liver problems

You will probably get only one or two of these side effects.

Maybe none at all.

Cyclophosphamide

is also called Cytoxan or CTX.

It can be given as either a pill or an IV shot.

CTX is one of a group of medicines called alkylating agents.

It acts by changing the way important molecules are shaped,

especially the DNA in cells that are growing fast.

CTX can cause one serious side effect.

It is called hemorrhagic cystitis.

CTX can hurt your bladder and make it bleed.

If your urine is pink or red

or if it hurts when you pass urine,

call your doctor.

You can help prevent this by

drinking lots of water while taking CTX.

Other side effects that CTX can cause are:

1. bone marrow depression
2. loss of appetite and nausea and vomiting
3. hair loss
4. sore mouth
5. diarrhea

You will probably get only one or two of these side effects.
Maybe none at all.

Bis-chloroethyl-nitrosourea

is also called carmustine or BCNU.

It can only be given as an IV shot.

BCNU does not belong to any special group of medicines

but it acts a lot like the ones in the alkylating agent group.

BCNU acts by changing

the way important molecules are shaped,

especially DNA in cells that are growing fast.

Side effects that BCNU can cause are:

1. bone marrow depression

2. nausea and vomiting

3. a burning feeling in the vein when you get the shot

You will probably have only one or two of these side effects.

The medicines explained here

are the ones that are now being used

to treat leukemia.

New medicines are being developed,

and it is not impossible

that you will be given a medicine

that isn't mentioned in this book.

If you are, you can use the next page

to write about it.

Ask your doctor if it is like

any of the other medicines on these pages.

That may help you understand it better.

And be sure to make a list of its common side effects.

You might also want to use these pages

to list the medicines you take

to treat other problems—

like antibiotics for infections—

that are related to your having leukemia.

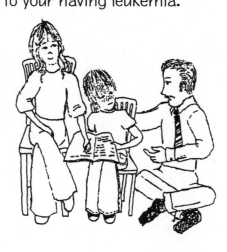

❋ NEW MEDICINES ❋

❋ NEW MEDICINES ❋

★Central Venous Catheters

Many of the medicines you need

to treat leukemia or its complications

need to be given as shots into a vein (IV).

So do blood transfusions (see pages 177-187)

and bone marrow transplants (see pages 188-198).

Also, if you get too nauseated to eat regular food,

you may need to be given liquid IV "food"

until you can eat again.

And many of the blood tests you will need to have

involve getting blood out of a vein.

After a while, people with leukemia

can start feeling like pincushions.

So, doctors figured out a way to do all this

that lets people with leukemia feel like people,

not like pincushions.

The way they do this is by using something called

a "central venous catheter" or CVC.

It can also be called a "central line," a "port"

or a "right atrial catheter."

The right atrium is a part of your heart.

Your heart (see page 19) is like a power plant

with four rooms, or chambers, in it.

Your veins, the roads that carry your blood to your heart,

enter your heart at the right atrium.

From there, your blood goes to the right ventricle,

which pushes it up into your lungs,

where your RBCs pick up a fresh supply of oxygen.

Then your blood goes to the chambers

on the left side of your heart,

which pushes it out into your arteries,

the roads to your body's cells.

A catheter is a soft plastic tube.

It's hollow like a straw but also bendable,

like spaghetti cooked half-way.

So a central venous catheter is a tube

with one end resting in the right atrium of your heart.

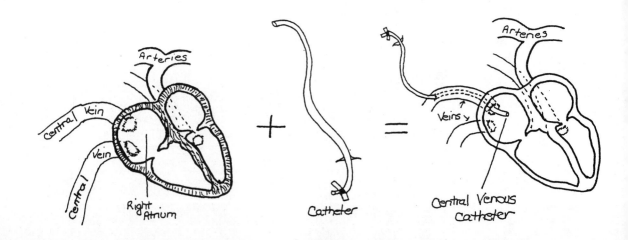

But where is the rest of the tube?

Most of it is in one of the large—or central—veins

that leads into your heart.

These veins are very big

and have plenty of room for a catheter inside them.

The other end of the tube

either comes out through the skin of your chest

or just ends at your skin.

depending on the kind of catheter that is used.

It's also the part that will be used

to give you the things you need

that must be given into a vein

without having to give you a shot each time.

The central venous catheter

(or CVC or central line)

takes the place of a lot of shots.

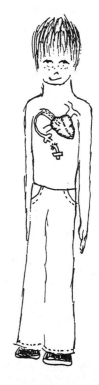

The CVC is put in place

by a surgeon.

Surgeons are doctors who do operations,

and it takes an operation to put in a CVC.

Operations can be painful,

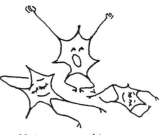

sleepy nerves

so the first thing that will happen when you have this operation

is that you will be given something so you don't feel pain.

You might be given a numbing medicine, such as EMLA,

to make the nerves in the area where the surgeon will work

fall sound asleep, like in a bone marrow test.

Or you might be given a medicine that makes <u>you</u> fall asleep,

and you'll sleep right through the whole procedure.

The kind of anesthesia—

or "no pain" medicine—that you receive

will depend on what you, your parents and your doctors

think is best for you.

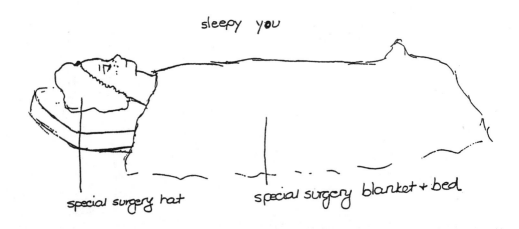

sleepy you

special surgery hat   special surgery blanket + bed

Once you are feeling no pain,

the surgeon will make two cuts in your skin.

One will be near your right shoulder,

over the spot where your CVC will go into your vein.

The other will be in the middle of your chest

where the catheter will either come out of your body

or where it will stop just under your skin.

Through those two cuts,

the surgeon will put the CVC in place.

Once it's there, the surgeon has to make sure

it stays where it's supposed to.

Surgeons do that by sewing, or stitching,

the catheter to the vein (where it goes in)

and to your skin (where it comes out or where it ends).

The only stitches you will see

will be the ones on your skin.

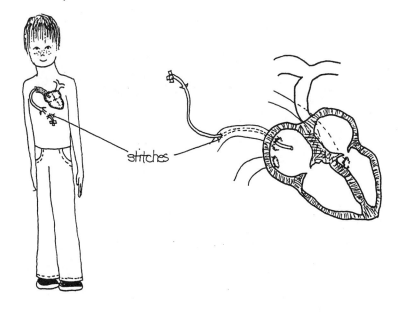

stitches

When the operation is over,

you will have two bandages.

There will be a small one near your right shoulder

and a big one on your chest,

over the spot where the CVC is.

The skin under these bandages

may be kind of sore for a few days,

the way the skin near any cut is sore at first.

The small cut near your shoulder will heal quickly.

The one where the catheter comes out or ends

will take many weeks to heal completely.

That's because the inside of your skin

has to kind of glue itself to the catheter

so that the CVC won't fall out

when the stitches are removed.

But you won't have to wait until the

stitches come out

to use the catheter.

It will be ready for action right away!

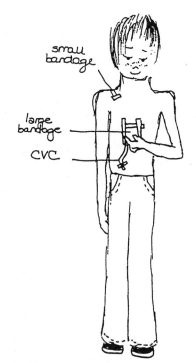

The first thing you'll notice about it

is that your arms are free again,

even when you're getting something IV.

The second thing you'll notice is that

you're not getting very many shots anymore.

That's because all the stuff you used to get as an IV

can now all be given into your CVC.

And usually blood can be taken out of it

when you need a blood test.

When you go home with your CVC

you'll be able to do everything you did before,

except for contact sports such as football or wrestling.

But gentler sports are safe.

Your catheter will be hidden under your clothes,

so no one will know you have it

(unless you want to show it to them).

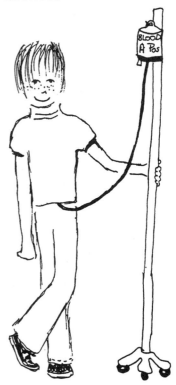

If your CVC is to stay in place for a long time,

it needs to be taken care of every day.

In the hospital, your nurses will do your catheter care.

But at home, you and your family will need to do it.

There are two goals in catheter care:

keeping the catheter clean

and keeping the catheter open.

It is kept clean by changing the bandage often.

It is kept open by

putting a medicine called heparin

into the catheter.

Catheter care is not hard to do,

and your nurses will teach you all how to do it

until you are as good at it as they are.

And CVCs that end right under your skin

don't need much care at all.

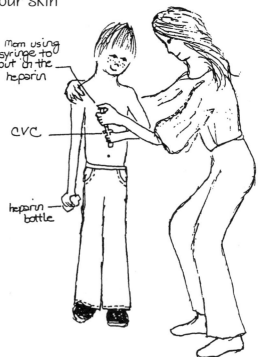

Mom using syringe to put in the heparin

cvc

heparin bottle

★ Spinal Taps

CNS leukemia (see pages 109-111)

can happen in both ALL and AML.

For this reason, early in the treatment of ALL,

medicine may be put in the CSF

to kill any blasts that might be hiding there

to try to prevent CNS leukemia later on.,

Or medicine might be put there

if you develop CNS leukemia.

The medicine has to be put where it's needed,

because it can't get to the spinal fluid any other way.

CSF is very snobby and doesn't mix much with blood.

The way the medicine, usually methotrexate

but sometimes Ara-C

or hydrocortisone (a cousin of prednisone)—

or a combination of two or more of those medicines—

is put into the spinal fluid

is by a procedure called a spinal tap.

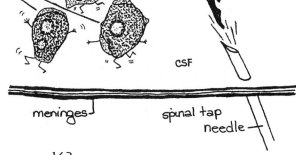

scared blasts

CSF

CSF

meninges

spinal tap needle

MTX

The spinal tap (also called lumbar puncture or LP)

is done either at the hospital or at the clinic.

You'll have some EMLA put on in advance, so it won't hurt.

You will lie down on your side on a table

or you may be asked to sit on the edge of the table.

You will have to pull up your shirt and lower your pants a little.

The doctor will ask you to curl up your body

by bringing your knees up to your chest if you're lying down

or sort of almost (but not quite) diving off the table

if you're sitting.

Your nurse will probably help you stay in this position.

That's because the more curled up you are,

and the stiller you are,

the easier it is for the doctor to work.

The doctor will stand behind you.

You will be prepped in about the same way as for a bone marrow.

The doctor will wear gloves and put towels on you

and wipe off your back with an antiseptic to kill germs.

The doctor will feel your back

for the very best place to put the needle in.

You won't feel much.

Maybe the scratchiness of the sponge used to wipe your back.

Maybe the coldness of the antiseptic.

Maybe a funny feeling of hot or cold in your legs

when the medicine is put in.

That's about it.

your position
(seen by the doctor)

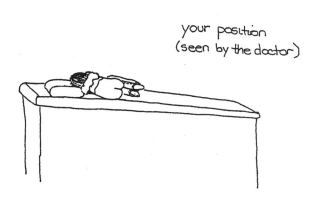

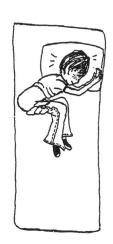

your
position

(seen from
the ceiling)

doctor, with gloves on
filling syringe with
xylocaine

medical student
holding bottle
of xylocaine

sterile
towel

your back,
with antiseptic
on it.

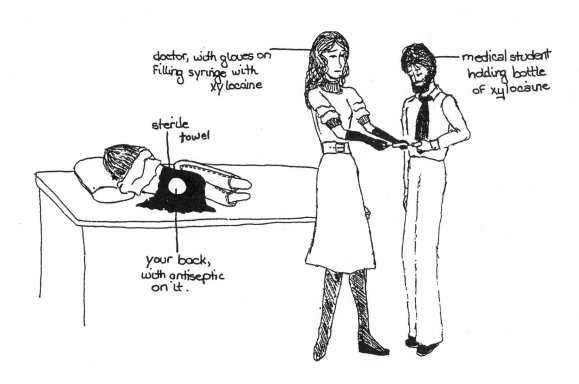

When your nerves have gotten very sleepy,

the doctor will take a special needle

(which has two parts, like the bone marrow needle)

and slide it past the sleepy nerves

through the meninges

and into the space where the CSF is found.

The doctor can tell when he or she is in the right place

because CSF—which looks just like water—

will begin to drip out of the hollow needle.

Sometimes the doctor will measure the pressure of the CSF

with a thing that looks like a big thermometer.

If you have CNS leukemia, the pressure will be high.

Then the doctor will let an exact amount of CSF

drop out into test tubes.

The doctor will measure the CSF pressure again.

After that, the medicine will be put in.

That can feel funny,

but it doesn't hurt.

When the medicine is all in, the needle will come out.

You'll feel a bandage being put on.

You'll be asked to stay lying down for a while

to try to keep you from getting a headache.

Sometimes people get headaches after spinal taps.

After a while you can go, depending on how you feel.

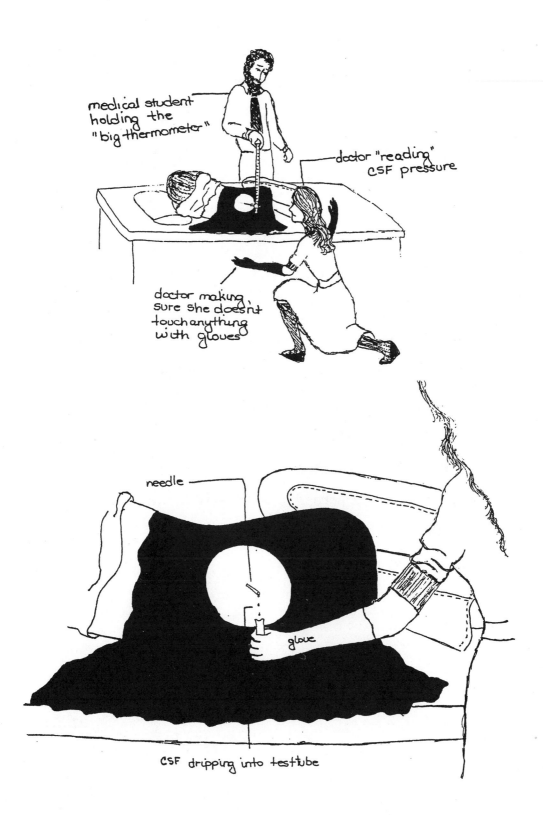

But the doctors can't go.

They have to look at your spinal fluid

to see if it's as clear as it should be.

If it's cloudy, it has too many cells.

They'll look at it under a microscope, too,

because there can still be too many cells

even when the CSF looks clear.

That way they can count the cells

and find out exactly what those cells are.

If there are any blasts, they will see them.

Other measurements will be done on your CSF,

like finding out how much sugar is there

and how much protein.

All of these measurements help doctors learn

if your leukemia has spread to your nervous system

and whether the treatment is working.

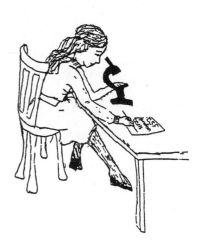

★Radiation Therapy

Radiation therapy is another form of treatment

used in leukemia and other cancers.

Radiation therapy is sort of like strong, smart, magic rays—

and best of all, radiation therapy doesn't hurt!

Radiation therapy is smart

because it can be aimed exactly at a small space

called a "field"

where a whole bunch of cancer cells are living together.

When there are many blasts in a small space,

radiation is often the best way to kill just those blasts

without hurting the nearby normal cells too much.

There are two places blasts can go

where radiation therapy really works well.

One is when blasts hide in the meninges,

in CNS leukemia.

The other is when blasts hide in the testes.

(Rarely, blasts can hide in other parts of the body

and radiation therapy can be helpful then, too.)

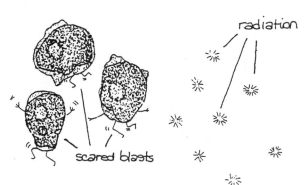

scared blasts

radiation

When radiation therapy is used for people with leukemia,

it's most often aimed at blasts

that might be hiding in the meninges,

to prevent CNS leukemia from ever happening.

In ALL, cranial radiation to prevent CNS leukemia

is usually done during the consolidation phase of treatment

if your leukemia is slow to get better from chemotherapy.

In AML, when needed, cranial radiation to prevent CNS leukemia

is also done early in treatment.

This special form of radiation therapy

is called cranial radiation,

and only your head is radiated.

Doctors have another word for head.

They call it a cranium.

So cranial radiation just means

radiation therapy to your head.

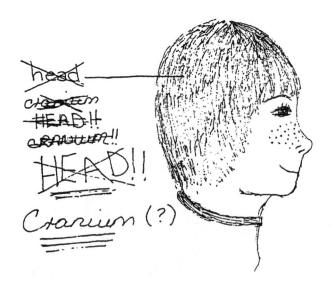

Whether you have ALL or AML,

if you get CNS leukemia

or if you have CNS leukemia

at the time your leukemia is diagnosed,

you will probably have radiation therapy

to both your cranium and your spine (backbone).

This is because both your brain

and the big nerves (spinal cord)

that connect your brain to the rest of you

are surrounded by CSF and covered by meninges.

If blasts show up in your CSF,

all of your meninges, not just the part around your brain,

needs to be treated.

Your brain and spinal cord are squishy parts.

The bones of your cranium and spine protect them.

So what do you think this kind of radiation therapy is called?

"Craniospinal," of course.

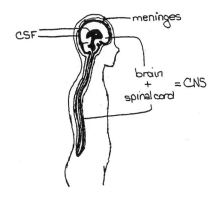

Some people think that radiation therapy

sounds scary and awful.

It's not really so bad.

For one thing, it doesn't hurt at all.

For another, it doesn't take very long.

Mostly what it does is to kill blasts.

The amount of radiation used is carefully figured out

so that it is enough to kill blasts

but not enough to kill the normal cells living nearby.

Luckily, normal cells are a lot tougher than blasts.

Normal cells might get sick for a while

but they almost always get better.

The cells that grow hair get the sickest,

so your hair will usually fall out.

Sometimes people get a little nauseated.

You might feel sleepier than usual

for a few months after your treatments are finished.

Rarely, radiation therapy to the cranium can cause cataracts,

which are like tiny blinders inside the eye.

You can help prevent this problem

by staying very still during your treatments.

Your first visit to the radiation therapy place

is called the "simulation," or just the "sim."

If you have ever played a computer game about Sims,

you already know what a sim is—

something that is almost like the real thing.

At the sim, you will meet some important people:

the special doctor, called a radiation oncologist,

who will be in charge of your treatments;

and the radiotherapists who will give you your treatments.

You will probably have your head measured

with a funny-looking thing called a caliper.

You'll go into the simulation room

and lay down on the simulation table,

so you can see what the room looks like and the table feels like.

You'll have x-rays taken of the fields to be irradiated

(you can practice not moving while this is done).

If you are having cranial radiation only,

a special "immobilizer" mask may be made

just for you

an immobilizer mask, from the side
(there's room inside for you + a headrest)

that will help you not move your head during the treatments.

(The masks are cool—they look like space alien faces.)

This is all a sim, a practice, to get you and everyone else

ready for your treatments.

Then, your appointments will be made

and your treatments will be set up to begin a day or two later.

All of your treatments will be pretty much the same.

You'll go into the treatment room.

If you're having cranial radiation,

you'll lie down on your back on the treatment table.

If you have a space alien mask, it will be put on

and attached to a special head rest.

You won't be able to see out of the mask

but you'll be able to breathe and hear just fine.

The radiotherapist may draw dots on your mask

or on your head if your treatment center doesn't use masks.

The dots mark exactly where the radiation should go.

If you're having craniospinal radiation it's pretty much the same,

except you'll lie on your tummy,

your mask will be on the back of your head

(if your treatment center uses them),

and you will get some extra dots or lines on your back.

Whichever kind of radiation therapy you're getting,

your job is the same: to not move.

The mask helps you do your job.

Sometimes straps buckled around you can help.

And if you're just a naturally wiggly

active person you might get some medicine

that would make you too sleepy to move.

Then, when you're all still and ready,

a bright light will come out of the machine

and shine on the part of you where the radiation will go.

radiation therapy machine

TV camera

you, in space alien mask
on comfortable table +
special headrest

When you are quiet and the machine has been aimed,

everyone but you will leave the room.

They will go into another room

where the controls to the machine are located.

But don't worry about being alone.

There's a TV camera in your room

and everyone is watching you on TV.

You—a TV star!

There's also a microphone and speakers

so you can hear and talk to everyone else.

Then you'll be given your treatment,

but the only way you will know that

is when the machine makes a buzzing noise.

No shots or anything like that.

Then the radiotherapist will come back

and move the machine to a different position.

(This may happen a couple of times.)

When the radiotherapist moves the machine away,

you're all finished for that day.

All of your treatments will be just like the first,

with both sides of your head being treated each time.

You can invite whoever is with you to watch you on TV

if your doctor says it's OK.

And you can ask to see the control room

where everyone else goes when you get your treatments.

Another time radiation therapy might be used

is if you get leukemia in your testes,

again because there are many blasts in a small space.

The side effects you might have if your testes are irradiated

are not the same as those from cranial radiation.

Often, with radiation therapy,

the skin that is in the way of the radiation

gets red and irritated—like a sunburn.

This can happen when testes are irradiated.

And there may be another side effect,

but you won't notice it until you grow up.

Your testes are where the special cells grow

that, when you're ready, help you have children.

If these cells are badly hurt by the radiation

it may not be possible for you to create children later on.

Nobody feels very good about taking a chance like that.

And, if it has to be done,

everyone hopes that when you grow up you will understand

how very much <u>you</u> mattered

for this decision to be made.

It's important for you to know, though,

that you will still be able to be a parent.

Lots of people can't create children from their

own bodies, but they can, and do,

have wonderful families.

★Blood Transfusions

Blood transfusions are often important

for people with leukemia.

So you should know

something about them.

To begin with,

blood that is used for transfusions

is given by healthy people who are called donors.

A donor usually gives

about a pint of blood at one time.

The blood can be used right away,

or, if it is kept cold,

blood can be used up to three weeks

after it is donated.

It is stored in a special place

called a blood bank.

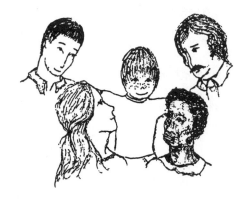

Blood, as you know,

is made up of many parts.

Whole blood, which contains all the different parts,

is usually not used

except for people who have lost a lot of blood.

Those patients need <u>all</u> the different things

in the donor's blood.

But most patients with leukemia

don't need whole blood.

Usually, only one part of their blood is missing—

like RBCs are missing in anemia

or platelets are missing in thrombocytopenia.

It makes a lot of sense

to separate all the different things in blood.

That way, blood from one donor

can help more than one patient.

The red cells can be given to a patient with anemia.

The platelets can be given to another patient

who has thrombocytopenia.

It makes a lot of sense,

and it's exactly what doctors do.

Usually, your transfusions will have only the part of blood

that <u>you</u> need.

What happens during a blood transfusion

is the same whether you're getting whole blood

or just one part (component).

A plastic bag

that contains blood chosen especially for you

is hung upside down at the top of a tall pole.

A long, skinny tube is connected

to the blood at one end

and to you at the other.

Since blood has to go directly into your veins

if it's to do any good,

you will have to have an IV needle in one of your veins

or your CVC will be used.

The blood is allowed to flow into your body slowly.

That way, if any problems occur,

the transfusions can be stopped

before you get very much

of the donor blood.

Even though problems don't come up

very often,

no one wants to take any chances with you.

If you need a blood transfusion,

it might be a good idea to

bring something to do

while the blood drips in.

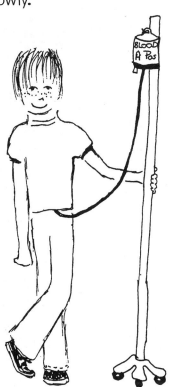

Blood transfusions,

like almost everything else in medicine,

can cause problems of their own.

For this reason, they're never used

unless they are really necessary.

They can cause two main kinds of problems.

One is that if the donor had a disease,

such as hepatitis (a liver disease)

or HIV (a T-cell disease)

when he or she gave the blood,

the germs that caused the disease may still be in the blood.

So you could get the disease.

No one wants this to happen.

Donors are chosen who appear to be healthy,

but sometimes a donor has a disease

and doesn't know it.

And the doctor doesn't know it.

So all donated blood is screened for these diseases.

But no matter how careful everyone is,

there is always the very small risk

of spreading a disease by

transfusing blood.

It almost never happens.

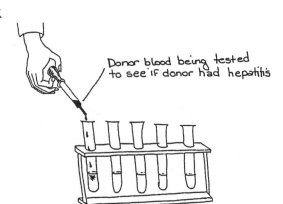

Donor blood being tested
to see if donor had hepatitis

The second type of problem

is harder to describe and explain.

It happens when your own immune system

treats the transfused blood as a foreign invader

and even tries to destroy it.

When you were very young,

the job of your immune system was to figure out

exactly what is <u>you</u> and what isn't.

Once it has figured you out,

for the rest of your life

your immune system will be on guard

against things in your body that are not like the rest of you.

So if your immune system

tries to destroy transfused blood,

it's just doing what it's supposed to do—

and you can't really blame it.

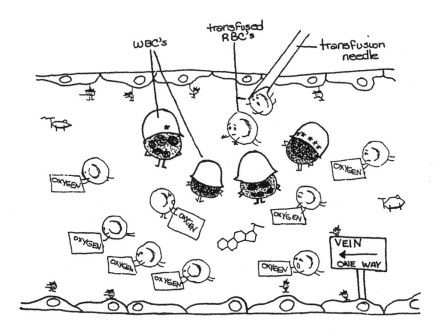

Friends?
or
Foes?

Luckily, scientists have learned a lot

about how your immune system works.

They learned that all the cells in your body

have little markers on them,

and the markers are called antigens.

Your immune system memorizes which antigens are yours,

and when it sees a cell with your antigens on it,

that cell is left alone.

But if it spies a cell

with antigens on it that are different from yours,

it will try to destroy that cell.

B-lymphocytes will make antibodies

that attach to the foreign antigens

and warn other cells that this is an enemy.

T-lymphocytes will organize other cells,

and all will work together to destroy the foreign cell.

This happens even when the foreign cell

was put there on purpose to help you,

as in a blood transfusion.

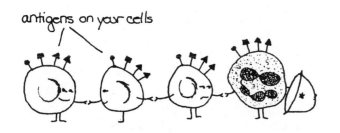

antigens on your cells

antigens on a foreign cell

But if your immune system sees a foreign cell

that has many of your antigens on it,

it will leave that cell alone,

just as it leaves your cells alone.

So a donor's blood is always tested

to see what antigens are on its cells,

and the blood that is given to you

will be as much like yours as possible.

Certain antigens are on red cells.

The most important of these

are called A and B.

Let's say that your blood is type A

(your blood cells have antigen A on them).

If you are given blood that is also type A,

your immune system will leave the new cells alone.

If you are given type B blood

(if the RBCs have B antigen on them),

your immune system will destroy the new cells.

You could also be given type O blood,

which means that the RBCs have neither A nor B antigens,

and your immune system will usually leave these cells alone.

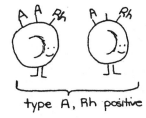

type A, Rh positive

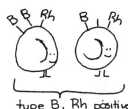

type B, Rh positive

type AB, Rh pos

type O, Rh pos

Another antigen that can be found on red cells is the Rh antigen.

If your RBCs have Rh antigen on them,

they are called Rh-positive, or just positive.

If your RBCs don't have the Rh antigen on them,

they are called Rh-negative, or just negative.

The most important antigens

in transfusing either whole blood or just red cells

are the A, B and Rh antigens.

Unless your blood is type O negative,

your RBCs will have one or more of these antigens.

And no matter what your blood type is,

the closer the match

between your blood and the donor's blood,

the fewer problems you will have.

Before you get a blood transfusion,

a little bit of your blood

will be mixed with the donor blood

to make sure they get along.

This is called a cross match.

It takes a while, at least an hour,

for the right blood to be chosen for you,

but it's worth the wait.

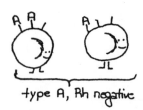
type A, Rh negative

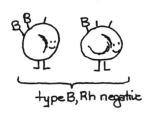
type B, Rh negative

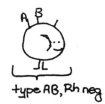
type AB, Rh neg

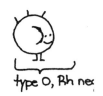
type O, Rh neg

If you have any of the following symptoms
while you are getting a blood transfusion,
you may be having a transfusion reaction:

1. skin rash and itching

2. fever

3. nausea and vomiting

4. a feeling that someone is sitting on your chest

5. yellow jaundice

6. low back pain

Luckily, transfusion reactions hardly ever happen.
But if you have any of these feelings,
tell the nurse or doctor right away.

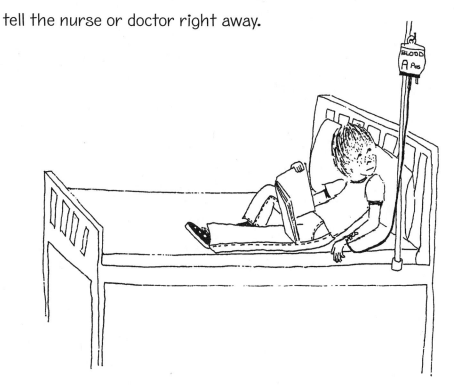

Transfusion of platelets

is a little more complicated.

These cells have antigens called

HL-A (histocompatibility) antigens

on their surfaces.

There are many different HL-A antigens,

and it's often hard

to find a donor who matches you exactly.

If you don't need transfusions

of platelets very often,

an exact match usually isn't necessary.

If an exact match can be found for you,

these cells will be used for transfusions.

HL-A antigens are also important

in bone marrow transplant procedures,

which we will talk about soon.

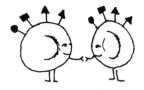

It's hard for anyone to predict

whether you will need many transfusions

or only a few.

Even so, you, your family, and your friends

know just how important it is

to have blood waiting for you in the blood bank

when you need it.

Blood for transfusions

can only come from people—

people who care about other people.

If it's possible,

you might want to ask your relatives and friends

to donate their blood to the blood bank.

In a way, it will replace the blood given to you.

The people who care about you

often feel frustrated and helpless.

They don't think they can do much to help you.

Tell them that donating blood to the blood bank

is one way they can help a lot.

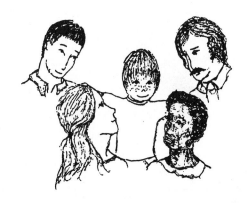

★Bone Marrow Transplants

The goal of most methods of treatment

is to destroy as many blasts as possible

without hurting normal cells too much.

If you were given enough chemotherapy

or radiation therapy

to destroy, for sure, every blast in your body,

your normal bone marrow cells

would probably be destroyed, too.

That wouldn't help you.

But what if a way were figured out

to give you new, healthy bone marrow

after your bone marrow had been destroyed?

Marrow from someone else,

someone who doesn't have leukemia.

There is a way to do this.

It's called a bone marrow transplant.

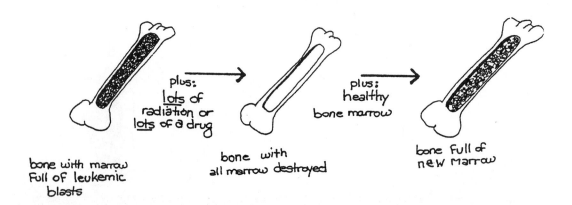

plus:
lots of
radiation or
lots of a drug

plus:
healthy
bone marrow

bone with marrow
full of leukemic
blasts

bone with
all marrow destroyed

bone full of
new marrow

The idea behind bone marrow transplants

is not hard to understand.

It is to destroy the bone marrow—

normal cells as well as blasts—

and then to replace it with new marrow.

It's easy to destroy bone marrow.

The transplant operation, as you will learn,

is not difficult to do.

This operation is now being done in several medical centers

for the treatment of leukemia.

Long remissions, even cures, have been made possible

by using bone marrow transplants.

However, there are problems that can make

bone marrow transplants both difficult and dangerous.

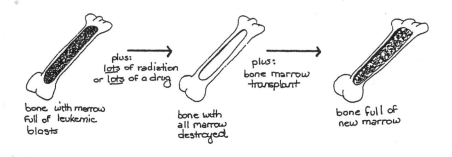

plus:
lots of radiation
or lots of a drug

plus:
bone marrow
transplant

bone with marrow
full of leukemic
blasts

bone with
all marrow
destroyed

bone full of
new marrow

One big problem is finding the right donor,

someone who will give you some of their bone marrow cells.

We have talked a little about HL-A antigens.

In transplants of any kind HL-A antigens are very important.

Unless both you and the donor have almost exactly the same

HL-A antigens on your cells, your immune system

will try to reject and destroy the donor cells.

It is the people in your close family—

especially your brothers and sisters—

whose HL-A antigens are most likely to match yours.

If you are an identical twin,

your twin brother or sister is the perfect donor.

His or her antigens are exactly like yours.

If you are not an identical twin,

your close family members can have their blood checked

to see if one of them has antigens enough like yours

to be your donor.

But even if you come from a large family,

it may not be possible to find the right donor for you

among your family.

If that happens, a search will be made to find

someone who is a match, even if they're not related to you.

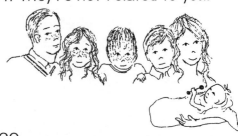

Another big problem is that your bone marrow must be destroyed

two or three weeks before you have the transplant.

This time is needed to turn your immune system off

so that it won't try to destroy the new bone marrow cells.

This period is dangerous for you because

you would have no defenses at all against infections.

For this reason you have to stay in the hospital,

in a special room,

away from anyone who might have an infection.

This isolation—keeping you away from other people—

is done to protect you.

Antibiotics, blood transfusions and isolation

can all help to get you safely through this time.

But you have to be ready to spend a few weeks

without as many visitors as usual.

Different transplant centers have different rules about isolation.

In some, careful handwashing is all your visitors need to do.

In others, even doctors, nurses and parents

will have to put on special clothes and masks

before they can come into your room.

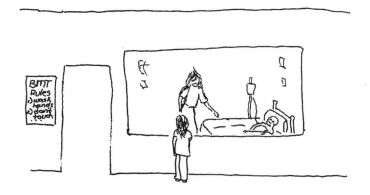

If you and your doctors decide

that a bone marrow transplant is the right treatment for you

and the right donor is found for you,

your bone marrow will be destroyed

with total body irradiation (TBI), with medicines or with both.

Then you will spend a few weeks in isolation.

You will get more medicines during this time

to shut down your immune system (immunosuppression).

The day you have the transplant,

the donor will be taken to the operating room.

She or he will be either put to sleep

or given lots of numbing medicine into the spine,

like in a spinal tap.

Then, when it won't hurt the donor,

many bone marrow aspirations

will be taken from the back of the donor's hip bone

(but there will usually be only one or two needle marks

on each side of the donor's hips).

This bone marrow will be checked by the doctor

and then it will be given to you

through an IV needle, like a blood transfusion.

The bone marrow cells will find their way

into the center of your bones

and will—everyone hopes—

start to grow there.

Your part of the transplant is easy.

Your donor may be a little sore, though.

Imagine having many bone marrow tests

all at the same time,

and you will know what your donor feels like.

Bone marrow is a very special gift.

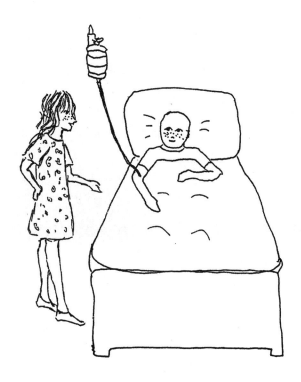

After the transplant,

you will have to go back into isolation.

You will be watched carefully

in case your body rejects the new cells.

There is still the problem of infection,

especially with a virus called CMV that almost everyone has

but that only bothers people

whose immune systems aren't working well.

Luckily, there is a good medicine to treat CMV.

And there is a new problem.

The new bone marrow cells

used to be part of the donor's immune system.

When they were still in the donor's body,

these same cells would help destroy foreign invaders.

In your body, these cells might decide that

your own cells are foreign invaders,

and the new cells would then try to destroy your cells.

The new cells don't know they've been transplanted.

All they know is that when they see cells that

look foreign to them, they must destroy the strange cells.

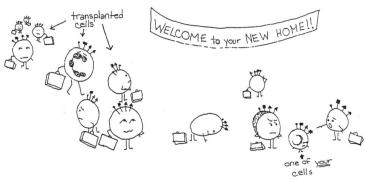

There is a name for this kind of problem.

It is called graft-versus-host disease

or GVHD for short.

It is common for people who get bone marrow transplants

to develop GVHD.

GVHD can be very mild or very serious.

Whether it happens at all

and how serious it is if it does happen

depend a lot on how well

your antigens and the donor's antigens match.

The symptoms and signs of GVHD

depend on how serious the disease is.

It can show up as just a skin rash

or it can go on to include blisters on the skin,

diarrhea, yellow jaundice

and even more risk of getting a very serious infection.

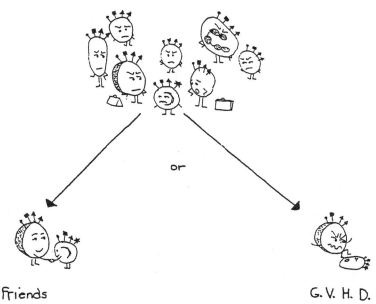

friends   G. V. H. D.

Once your doctors have decided

that your body likes its new bone marrow

and the new marrow is used to its new home,

you can leave your isolation room.

This is a very exciting day for everyone.

You can finally share

all the hugs and kisses you've been saving up.

Especially for your donor

if your donor is your relative or a friend.

You will be in a new remission.

Maybe you will have to take some medicines

and maybe not,

but you will still have to see your doctor often,

the same as with other remissions.

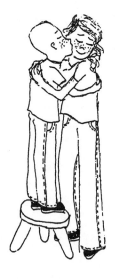

When a bone marrow transplant is successful,

it is a very effective treatment for leukemia.

But not every transplant is successful.

And the weeks of waiting and hoping

while you are still in isolation

can be hard for you and the people who love you.

For these reasons, the operation isn't done lightly.

Usually, bone marrow transplants are performed

only when your doctors think other forms of treatment

are no longer enough to keep your leukemia in control.

If you have ALL and are in remission

but have had several relapses in the past,

a bone marrow transplant might be offered.

If you have AML, a bone marrow transplant

could be offered sooner,

maybe while you're still in your first remission.

That's because medicines and radiation therapy

haven't worked as well with AML as with ALL.

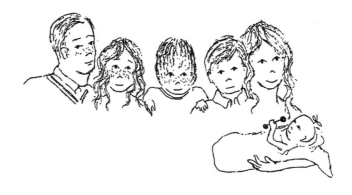

As doctors do more and more bone marrow transplants,

they are getting the experience they need

to treat the complications more effectively.

Even now, progress is being made.

Medicines like cyclosporin-A,

which makes the immune system less active,

are helping make GVHD a much less severe problem.

Medications like acyclovir and ganciclovir

are now available to fight some virus infections.

Doctors are learning more about HL-A antigens,

and they are able to make much better matches

between you and your donor.

Maybe someday you won't even need a donor.

Doctors are trying to find ways

to take your own bone marrow

when you're in remission,

treat it for any leftover leukemia cells,

and nurture it so that the healthy cells grow.

Then, if you start to have a relapse,

you can be given a transplant of your own marrow

and a lot of complications could be avoided.

Many problems remain, however, and much

needs to be learned

before it's as easy to <u>do</u> bone marrows

as it is to <u>think</u> about doing them.

★Immunotherapy

You have learned a lot about your immune system.

You have learned that its goal

is to protect your body from foreign invaders.

You have learned that it's made up of

many different kinds of cells (see pages 32-33),

and that these cells all have different jobs to do

in your body's defense.

You have learned how the cells of your immune system

can figure out which cells are yours and which are not,

depending on their antigens (see pages 182-186)

and what the different parts of the immune system do

when they run into cells with the wrong antigens.

Given all that you have learned

about what the immune system does,

you can probably guess what immunotherapy is.

Immunotherapy is a kind of treatment

designed to help your immune system

do a better job in fighting your leukemia.

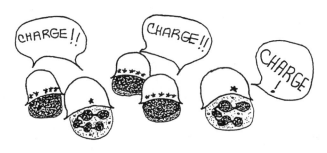

Often, by the time any cancer causes symptoms and signs,

the immune system just can't deal with it anymore.

There are simply too many malignant cells.

In leukemia, there is a double problem.

Not only are there too many malignant cells,

but these cells are the very ones your immune system needs

to do its work right.

Chemotherapy and radiation therapy can destroy

many of these malignant cells.

In fact, they may actually destroy enough malignant cells

so that your own immune system could destroy the rest

if it's working properly.

But, in leukemia, it usually isn't.

So, just at the exact moment when

your immune system has the chance

to destroy the remaining malignant cells,

it may not be able to.

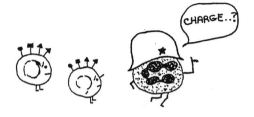

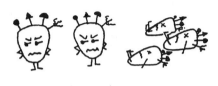

If your doctors want to help your immune system

get rid of your leftover malignant cells,

there are many ways they might go about it.

One thing they might try is to help your whole immune system

get more excited about doing its job.

There are substances that do this.

One is called granulocyte colony stimulating factor,

but since that's too much for anyone to say (including doctors)

it's just called GCSF.

Other substances can be certain antigens

or even germs that don't make you sick

but that do make your immune system especially active

against all kinds of foreign antigens.

The idea is that your immune system might also

become especially active

against the antigens on your leukemia cells.

Those antigens aren't exactly foreign,

but they are also not the same as the antigens

on your normal cells.

These substances, called BCG and MER,

have been found to work well against

some kinds of skin cancer.

But they don't work so well

against leukemia.

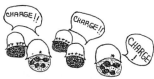

It may not be necessary to excite

the whole immune system

to create an effective kind of immunotherapy for leukemia.

Vaccinations, like the ones you had before you got leukemia

to protect you against diseases like tetanus and polio,*

work by just exciting a part of the immune system.

Vaccinations help your B-cells make antibodies

against the antigens on certain germs,

so if those germs ever show up again in your body

your immune system will destroy them

and you won't get sick.

Maybe a vaccine can be made against leukemia antigens.

Maybe, but it hasn't happened yet.

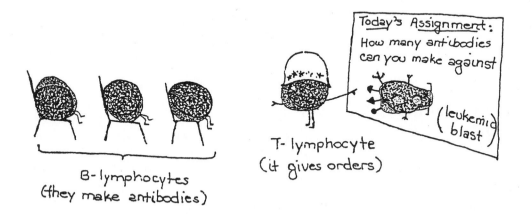

B- lymphocytes
(they make antibodies)

T- lymphocyte
(it gives orders)

Today's Assignment:
How many antibodies
can you make against

(leukemia
blast)

---

*Now that you have leukemia, you won't get any more vaccinations until your doctors think you are all better.

Antibodies might be helpful in another way.

Let's say that someone could find

a special malignant antigen on your blasts.

And let's say that the same antigen could be found

on the blasts of all the people who have

the same kind of leukemia you do.

It would then be possible to make an antibody

that would attach to only this antigen.

This antibody might be able to alert

the rest of the immune system,

which could then destroy the blast.

Or one of the medicines you take

to kill blasts

could be attached to this antibody.

The antibody would carry the medicine

right to its target: the blasts.

The medicine could do its blast-killing job better

while causing less damage to your normal cells.

This is being tried now in patients with some kinds of cancer.

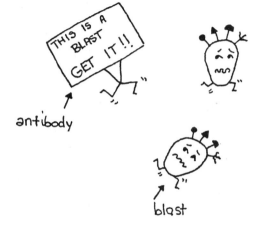

antibody

blast

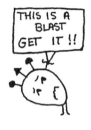

antibodies
attached to blasts

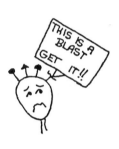

Other kinds of immunotherapy

using different parts of the immune system

are being, or have been, experimented with.

For example, some doctors have taken lymphocytes

and put them through special treatments

to make them into very nasty fighters,

kind of like "terminator" lymphocytes.

These killer cells are then injected into cancer patients,

where it is hoped they will mercilessly kill cancer cells.

It doesn't always work out, though.

Sometimes the killer lymphocytes are themselves destroyed

by the patient's immune system before they can do any good.

And sometimes the killer cells make the cancer patients sicker

by causing GVHD (see page 195).

Since putting whole cells into patients

can cause so much trouble,

other doctors are just injecting

the biochemical commands that lymphocytes make

such as interferon, interleukin,

transfer factor and immune-RNA.

These chemicals contain information

that the cells in your immune system

can use to do their job better.

It's sort of like learning from a book

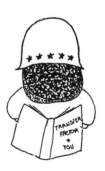

instead of from experience.

If you receive immunotherapy

as part of your treatment program,

you will probably get

one of the types described here.

You can also think of a bone marrow transplant

as a kind of immunotherapy

because it gives you a new healthy immune system

in addition to getting rid of blasts.

Doctors are excited about immunotherapy

because it offers both them and us

the possibility of finding treatments

for diseases that have no real treatment now

(like the common cold)—

as well as offering us all the possibility

that we can make the current treatment of leukemia

even more effective

than it already is.

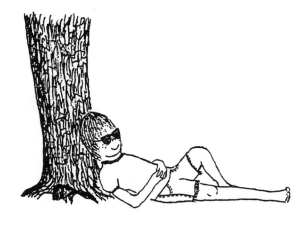

The Beginning

This book can't have an ending,

but like all books, it has to stop sometime.

Stopping isn't the same as ending.

First of all, the progress in treating and curing leukemia

hasn't ended.

New ideas are happening every day.

New clinical trials are beginning all the time.

Because of that, this book can only reflect

this moment in time.

It is meant to be your guide,

a help, a friend,

as you live through your days with leukemia.

Most of you who are now living with leukemia

will go on to live without it.

If you are one of these,

there can't possibly be enough room in this book

for all the pages of your life.

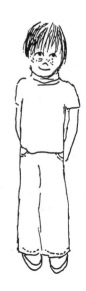

It will be up to you to write another book about you

and your life after leukemia.

We know how it should start:

"I . . . am very special."

You have to take it from there.

We don't know all that will be in your book

but we can guess about some things.

You may wonder all your life about why you ever had leukemia.

You may struggle with why you lived when others didn't,

but you don't need to feel guilty about being alive.

A whole bunch of people were hoping you would be,

most of whom you don't even know and never will.

You may feel that, being a leukemia survivor,

you always have to be a hero—

when all you have to be is a person.

You may never trust life to be as kind

as others do.

You may value life as few others can.

The challenge of surviving a disease

like leukemia is both a difficult and a

rewarding one.

All of us hope you have the chance

to meet this challenge,

a day at a time.

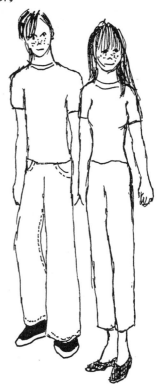

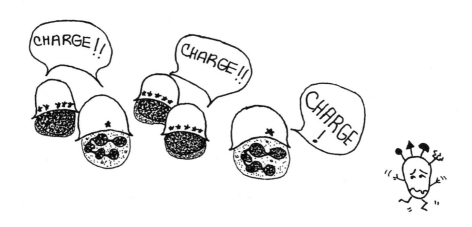

Additional Resources

When I first put this list together, there were very few sources of information just for children with leukemia or other cancers or for their families. More amazingly, the Internet didn't exist. Now there are great books available, wonderful booklets, super community organizations, and terrific websites. If you want to, you can find enough information to fill up a whole house!

Some of the books on this list are old and may not be in print anymore, but I am listing my favorite ones anyway. These are not necessarily about leukemia but about the body, germs, DNA, emotions, and the cycles of life—so they continue to be of value, especially those written for children. They may be available in bookstores, your public library, your school library, or via dot.com bookstores. The newer books listed here, on the other hand, were written especially for the families and other caregivers of kids with leukemia, and some of the booklets were written for children with leukemia and other cancers. These are often available in technical bookstores, at dot.com bookstores, or direct from the publishers, as this book is.

More resources besides books are available for kids with leukemia and their families than there used to be. Many national organizations, usually with local chapters, exist to provide information and other kinds of help. The Internet is another source of both information and support. If you don't have a computer at home, your treatment center will likely have one you can use, or your local library, or your school.

As always, if anything you read or learn causes you to have questions (and I hope you have lots of questions), be sure to ask your doctor, nurse, patient educator, or child life specialist about them.

Books

Adams DW and Deveau EJ: *Coping With Childhood Cancer: Where Do We Go From Here?* Canada, Kinbridge, 1997.

Allison L: *Blood and Guts: A Working Guide to Your Own Insides.* Boston, Little, Brown and Company, 1976. For kids.

Berenstain S and Berenstain J: *The Berenstain Bears Go to the Doctor.* New York, Random House, 1981. For kids.

Berger M: *Germs Make Me Sick!* New York, Harper and Row, 1985. For kids.

Buscaglia L: *The Fall of Freddie the Leaf: A Story of Life for All Ages.* Thorofare, NJ, Slack, Inc., 1982. About the cycle of life.

Center for Attitudinal Healing: *There Is a Rainbow Behind Every Dark Cloud.* Tiburon, CA, Center for Attitudinal Healing, 1978. For kids and grownups.

Ciliotta C and Livingston C: *Why Am I Going to the Hospital?* Secaucus, NJ, Lyle Stuart, Inc., 1981. For kids.

Elting M: *The Macmillan Book of the Human Body.* New York, Macmillan Publishing Company, 1986. For kids.

Glasser RJ: *The Body Is the Hero.* New York, Random House, 1976. For teenagers and adults, about how the immune system works.

Grollman E: *Talking About Death.* New York, Dell Publishing Co., 1975. Rabbi Grollman's book is for children and grownups to read together.

Janes-Hodder H and Keene N: *Childhood Cancer: A Parent's Guide to Solid Tumor Cancers.* For those of you whose children may have cancers other than leukemia.

Keene N: *Childhood Leukemia: A Guide for Families, Friends and Caregivers.* Sebastopol, CA, O'Reilly & Associates, 1999.

Keene N, Hobbie W, and Ruccione K: *Childhood Cancer Survivors: A Practical Guide to Your Future.* Sebastopol, CA, O'Reilly & Associates, 2000. For survivors.

Keene N and Prentice R: *Your Child in the Hospital: A Guide for Parents.* Sebastopol, CA, O'Reilly & Associates, 1999.

Kubler-Ross E: *On Children and Death.* New York, Macmillan Publishing Company, 1985. For grownups.

Kushner HS: *When Bad Things Happen to Good People.* New York, Avon Books, 1981. For grownups.

LeShan E: *What Makes Me Feel This Way? Growing Up With Human Emotions.* New York, Collier Books, 1972. For kids.

Mayer M: *There's a Nightmare in My Closet.* New York, Dial Books for Young Readers, 1968. For kids who are scared of the dark . . . and of other things. A classic.

Mayle P: *Will I Go to Heaven?* New York, Corwin Books, 1976. For kids.

Nessem S and Ellis J: *Cancervive: The Challenge of Life After Cancer.* Boston, Houghton Mifflin Co., 1991. For survivors.

Thomas L: *Lives of a Cell: Notes of a Biology Watcher.* New York, Bantam Books, Inc., 1974. For teenagers and grownups, about . . . life!

Watson JD: *The Double Helix.* New York, New American Library, Inc., 1968. For teenagers and grownups, about how scientists figured out what DNA did.

Booklets

American Cancer Society: *Back to School: A Handbook for Parents of Children With Cancer.* Call toll free: 1-800-ACS-2345 or www.cancer.org

American Cancer Society: *Back to School: A Handbook for Teachers of Children With Cancer.* Call toll free: 1-800-ACS-2345 or www.cancer.org

American Cancer Society: *What Happened to You Happened to Me.* Call toll free: 1-800-ACS-2345 or www.cancer.org

American Cancer Society: *When Your Brother or Sister Has Cancer.* Call toll free: 1-800-ACS-2345 or www.cancer.org

Cagelosi J, Miceli T, Siede B, and Fineberg B: *The Radiation Therapy Coloring Book: A Child's View of RT and an Activity Book.* New Orleans, Oschner Medical Foundation, 1999.

Leukemia and Lymphoma Society of America: *Emotional Aspects of Childhood Leukemia: A Handbook for Parents.* 1998. Call: (212) 573-8484 or www.leukemia.org

Meadows AT and Fenton JG: *Taking Charge of Your Health: A Guide to Medical Follow-up for Young Adults Who Had Cancer in Childhood.* Philadelphia, Children's Hospital of Philadelphia, 1995.

National Cancer Institute (NCI): *Cancer Survivorship: An Annotated Bibliography.* NIH Publication No. 91-3173, 1990. For all NCI publications, you can reach them at www.nci.nih.gov

National Cancer Institute (NCI): *Chemotherapy and You: A Guide to Self-Help During Cancer Treatment.* National Institutes of Health (NIH) Publication No. 99-1136, 1999.

National Cancer Institute (NCI): *Facing Forward: A Guide for Cancer Survivors.* NIH Publication No. 90-2424, 1990.

National Cancer Institute (NCI): *Managing Your Child's Eating Problems During Cancer Treatment.* NIH Publication No. 94-2038, 1994.

National Cancer Institute (NCI): *Radiation Therapy and You: A Guide To Self-Help During Cancer Treatment.* NIH Publication No. 98-2227, 1998.

National Cancer Institute (NCI): *Taking Part in Clinical Trials: What Cancer Patients Need to Know.* NIH Publication No. 98-4270, 1998.

National Cancer Institute (NCI): *Taking Time: Support for People With Cancer and the People Who Care About Them.* NIH Publication No. 97-2059, 1997.

National Cancer Institute (NCI): *What You Need to Know About Leukemia.* NIH Publication No. 95-3775, 1994.

National Cancer Institute (NCI): *When Someone in Your Family Has Cancer.* NIH Publication No. 96-2685, 1995.

National Cancer Institute (NCI): *Young People With Cancer.* NIH Publication No. 93-2378, 1988.

National Coalition for Cancer Survivorship: *Teamwork: The Cancer Patient's Guide to Talking With Your Doctor.* National Coalition for Cancer Survivorship (NCCS), 1991. Call (877) NCCS-YES or (877) 622-7937 or www.cansearch.org

Organizations—General Support and Information

American Cancer Society
  National Office
  1599 Clifton Road, NE
  Atlanta, GA 30329
  (800) ACS-2345
  www.cancer.org

Cancer Care
  275 Seventh Avenue
  New York, NY 10001
  (800) 813-HOPE or
  (212) 302-2400

Cancer Cured Kids
  P.O. Box 189
  Old Westbury, NY 11568
  (516) 484-8160

Cancer Kids
  P.O. Box 2715
  Waxahachie, TX 75168
  www.cancerkids.org

Cancervive
  6500 Wilshire Boulevard,
  Suite 500
  Los Angeles, CA 90048
  (310) 203-9232

Candlelighters Childhood Cancer
Foundation
  3910 Warner Street
  Kensington, MD 20895
  (800) 366-CCCF or
  (301) 962-3520
  www.candlelighters.org

Leukemia and Lymphoma Society
(formerly Leukemia Society of
America)
  733 Third Avenue
  New York, NY 10017
  (212) 573-8484
  www.leukemia.org

National Cancer Institute (NCI)
  Office of Cancer Communica-
  tions
  Cancer Information
  Clearinghouse
  9000 Rockville Pike
  Building 31, Room 10A-18
  Bethesda, MD 20205
  www.cancernet.nci.nih.gov

National Childhood Cancer
Foundation (NCCF)
  440 E. Huntington Drive
  Arcadia, CA 91066-6012
  (800) 458-NCCF
  Fax: (626) 447-6359
  www.nccf.org

National Coalition for Cancer
Survivorship (NCCS)
  1010 Wayne Avenue, Suite 770
  Silver Spring, MD 20910-5600
  (877) NCCS-YES or
  (877) 622-7937
  www.cansearch.org

Oranizations—Hair Loss, Facial Differences, and Learning Disabilities

Hip Hat
   3733 Shore Boulevard
   Oldsmar, FL 34677
   (877) HIP-HATS or
   (877) 447-4287
   Fax: (813) 314-0139
   www/hiphat.com

Learning Disabilities Association
   4156 Library Road
   Pittsburgh, PA 15234-1349
   (412) 341-1515

Let's Face It
   P.O. Box 29972
   Bellingham, WA 98228
   (360) 676-7325

Locks of Love
   160 S. Congress Avenue,
   Suite 104
   Palm Springs, FL 33416
   (888) 896-1588 or
   (561) 963-1677
   www.locksoflove.org

Organizations—Legal Rights

Cancer Legal Resource Center
   919 S. Albany Street
   Los Angeles, CA 90015-0019
   (213) 736-1455

Childhood Cancer Ombudsman's
Program
   P.O. Box 595
   Burgess, VA 22432
   Fax: (804) 580-2502 or
   (804) 580-2304

National Association of Protection
and Advocacy Systems
   900 2nd Street NE, Suite 211
   Washington, DC 20002
   (202) 408-9514

Organizations—Hospice

Children's Hospice International
   2202 Mt. Vernon Avenue,
   Suite 3C
   Alexandria, VA 22301
   (800) 24-CHILD

Additional Websites

Ask Noah About Cancer
www.noah-health.org

CancerSourceKids.com
www.CancerSourceKids.com

Children's Cancer Web—A Guide To Internet Resources for Childhood
Cancer
www.cancerindex.org/ccw

Kids Cancer Network
www.kidscancernetwork.org

Kid's Home At NCI
www.cancernet.nci.nih.gov/occdocs/kidshome.html

National Marrow Donor Program
www.marrow.org/index.html

National Office of Cancer Survivorship
www.dccps.nci.nih.gov/ocs

Oncolink
www.cancer.med.upenn.edu/disease

Outlook—Life Beyond Cancer
www.outlook-life.org

Squirrel Tales
www.squirreltales.com

Glossary of Words Not Defined in the Text

alkylating agents
  (*al'*-kill-ate-ting)

A group of medicines that can be used to treat many kinds of cancers, including leukemia. These medicines change the shapes of important molecules, especially DNA, in cells that are dividing rapidly.

antibiotics
  (ant-ty-by-*ah'*-ticks)

A group of medicines that can kill living things or stop them from growing. Some antibiotics kill bacteria, so these are used to treat infections. Others kill cancer cells, so they are used to help people with cancers.

antimetabolite
  (ant-ty-met-*tab'*-oh-lite)

A group of medicines that can be used to treat cancers and some other diseases. These medicines act by stopping cells from making DNA, so they can't divide.

bacteria
  (back-*tea'*-ree-ah)

Very small living beings made of just one cell, and that cell doesn't even have a proper nucleus. Bacteria are one kind of germ, and most of them are harmless. Some of them can cause diseases if they get inside our bodies.

benign
  (bee-*nine'*)

Good, not harmful.

chemicals
  (*keh'*-mick-calls)

Everything in the universe that you can touch is made of chemicals: stars, rocks, trees, frogs, and people.

diagnosis
  (dye-ahg-*know'*-sis)

The process of figuring out what disease a person has.

216

drug

A chemical, whether "natural" or manmade, that is used to treat or prevent diseases or to make the symptoms less serious. Because the word "drug" now has gotten a bad reputation due to illegal drugs, this book usually uses the word "medicine" instead.

enzyme
    (*ehn'*-zime)

A protein that helps a chemical reaction happen sooner or go faster than it would otherwise. Many medicines act by interfering with the body's own enzymes. Others are enzymes themselves.

fungus

One-celled living beings, most of which are harmless or even useful to people—such as the mushrooms we eat or the yeast we use to make bread. But some funguses, or fungi, can cause diseases if they get into our bodies.

glass slide

A small, thin, rectangular piece of clear glass that things are put on in order to look at them through a microscope.

hematocrit
    (hee-*mat'*-oh-krit)

A measurement of the percentage of whole blood that is made up of red blood cells.

hematology
    (hee-mah-*tah'*-la-gee)

The study of blood and diseases of the blood and blood-making organs.

hemoglobin
    (*hee'*-moh-glow-bin)

The stuff in red blood cells that gives them both their red color and their ability to carry oxygen.

histocompatibility antigens
    (*hiss'*-toe-come-pat-
    ah-*bill'*-it-tee)

"Histo" means tissue, which in doctor-talk is sort of a general word for flesh. "Compatible" means being able to get along. So this word refers to the antigens that can be looked at to tell if tissue from two different people will be able to live and grow together, as in a bone marrow transplant.

hormone	A chemical that is either produced by our bodies or that scientists can make in laboratories. Normally, hormones just keep our bodies running smoothly. When used in larger amounts to treat diseases, they are thought of as medicines.
identical twins	The kind of twins it is hard to tell apart unless you know them really well. They start out as just one cell but end up becoming two people.
infection	What happens when tiny living things, such as bacteria or viruses or fungi or parasites, get inside our bodies and make us sick.
ionizing radiation (*eye'*-oh-ny-zing)	Radiation that changes a chemical that has no electrical charge into one that does.
lymph (*limf*)	The liquid that is found in lymphatic vessels.
lymph node	A bunch of lymphocytes all in one place. Lymph nodes can become very large in certain diseases, but they are usually small and can barely be felt.
malignant (ma-*lig'*-nent)	Bad, harmful.
molecule (*ma'*-leh-kyool)	An itty-bitty bit of matter that is made up of even smaller bits called "atoms."
oncology (on-*kah'*-lah-gee)	The study of cancers.
oxygen (*ox'*-ih-jen)	A gas in the air we breathe that is necessary to maintain life for all animals on earth.
parasites (*pear'*-ah-sites)	Animals that must live inside other animals to survive and that often cause diseases for the animal they live in. Some parasites are tiny, consisting of only one cell. Others, like worms, can be much bigger.

RNA	A molecule very much like DNA that makes it possible for the ideas in DNA to be carried out.
scalpel	A special little knife doctors use to cut skin.
spleen	A big organ in the top of the belly on the left side. It helps the blood work right but can also be a place where cancer cells can get together in diseases like leukemia and lymphoma.
thymus gland (*thigh'*-muss)	A gland located in the upper front part of the chest, behind the breastbone. It is a place where T-cells grow up and learn how to do their jobs.
vinca alkaloids (*vink'*-ah *al'*-kah-loyds)	A group of medicines that can be used to treat cancers. They stop cells from dividing.
viruses (*vy'*-russ-says)	Very tiny things that are only really alive when they can infect living cells. Most of them are harmless, but some can cause diseases.
x-rays	A kind of radiation that can be used to take "pictures" of the insides of people, where light (another form of radiation and the kind we use to take snapshots) can't go.

Index

flu, viruses and, 51
friends, 118, 120-121
funguses, 33

G

ganciclovir (jan-sigh´-klow-veer), 198
gasoline, 50
GCSF (granulocyte colony stimulating factor), 201
general anesthesia, 75, 158
genes (jeans), 8, 45, 53
genetic (jeh-neh´-tick) factors, 44, 45
germs, 32
  blood transfusions and, 180
  infections and, 107-108
  skin and, 16
glands, 14
"goose bumps," 16
graft-versus-host disease (GVHD), 194-195, 198, 204
granisetron (gra-niss´-eh-tron) (Kytril), 128
granulocyte colony stimulating factor (GCSF), 201
granulocytes (gran´-you-low-sites), 32, 69, 102
  immature (im´-mat-cher), 60, 70
granulocytic (gran´-you-low-sit´-tick) leukemia, 56
GVHD (graft-versus-host disease), 194-195, 198, 204

H

hair loss, 125, 172
HCT (hematocrit [hee-mat´-oh-krit]), 68
headaches, 166
health educators, 119
heart, 19, 156
heart murmurs, 26, 27
heartburn, 126
hematocrit (hee-mat´-oh-krit) (HCT), 68
hematoma (hee-mah-toe´-mah), 103, 104
hemoglobin (hee´-mow-glow-bin) (HGB), 68
hemorrhagic (hem´-or-aj-ick) cystitis, 150
heparin (heh´-per-in), 162
hepatitis (heh-pah-tie´-tiss), 180
HGB (hemoglobin), 68
histocompatibility (hiss-toe-come-pat-ah-bill´-it-tee) (HL-A) antigens, 186, 190, 198
history, taking a, 62
HIV, 180
HL-A (histocompatibility) antigens, 186, 190, 198
hormones, 14, 24
hospice (hah´-spiss), 100
hydrocortisone (hi-drow-core´-tih-zone), 163

I

identical twins
  genes of, 45
  HL-A antigens and, 190
IM (intramuscular), 144, 146
immature (im´-mat-cher) cells, 70
immature granulocytes, 60, 70

immature lymphocytes, 70
immature monocytes, 70
"immobilizer" mask, 173, 174
immune (im´-yoon) system, 181-185, 199-205
immune-RNA, 204
immunologic (im´-you-no-lah´-jick) factors, 44, 54-55
immunology (im´-you-nah´-la-gee), 54
Immunosuppression (im-you-no-suh-preh´-shun), 192
immunotherapy (im´-you-no-thair´-ah-pea), 54, 137, 199-205
induction (in-duck´-shun) program, 91, 92
infections, 31, 106-108, 151, 194
intensification program, 95-96
interferon (in-ter-fear´-on), 204
interim maintenance program, 94
interleukin (in-ter-luke´-in), 204
Internet chat rooms, 133
interns, 120
intramuscular (in-trah-musk´-you-ler) (IM), 144, 146
intravenous (in-trah-vee´-nuss) (IV), 91, 140, 155, 161
"intuition," 113
investigational drugs, 87
isolation, bone marrow transplant and, 191, 192, 194
IV (intravenous), 91, 140, 155, 161

J

jaundice (jawn´-diss), 147

K

kidney problems, 112
Kytril (granisetron), 128

L

lab technicians (teck-nish´-shuns), 119
laxatives, 126
length of life, 131
leukemia (loo-key´-me-ah), 27, 41-114
  causes of, 43-44
  CNS, 109-111, 163, 166, 169, 170, 171
  complications of, 102-114
  diagnosing, 61-85
  kinds of, 56-60
  living with, 116-135
  meningeal, 109
  testicular, 113-114
  treatment for, 86-101, 136-153
leukemia cells, 57-58, 60, 109
leukocytes (loo´-koh-sites) (WBCs; white blood cells), 23, 25, 30, 31, 32-34, 36, 37, 38, 54, 56, 68, 69, 71, 106
leukopenia (loo-koh-pea´-knee-ah), 31
lightning, 50
liver, leukemic blasts and, 58
liver cancer, 53

liver damage, 146, 147, 148
LP (lumbar puncture), 164
lumbar puncture (LP), 164
lymph (limf) nodes, 38
   leukemic blasts and, 58
   lymphomas and, 52
lymphatic (lim-fat´-ick) vessels, 19
lymphoblasts (lim-foe´-blasts), 57-58, 60
lymphocytes (lim-foe´-sites), 33, 38, 69, 102, 204
   ALL and, 57-58
   atypical, 70
   immature, 70
   "terminator," 204
lymphocytic (lim-foe-sit´-ick) leukemia, 56
lymphoma (lim-foe´-mah), Burkitt's, 52

M

magnetic fields, 50
"maintenance," 94
maintenance program, 97
maintenance therapy, 96
malignant cells, 42, 46, 57-58
mask, immobilizer, 173, 174
maturation (mat-choo-ray´-shun), 38
measles, 106
medical students, 120
medical technicians, 119
meningeal (men-in-gee´-yall) leukemia, 109
meninges (men-in´-jeez), 109, 170
MER, 201
6-mercaptopurine (mer-cap-toe-pure-een)
   (6-MP), 147
metamyelocytes (met-ah-my´-ell-oh-sites), 70
methotrexate (meth-oh-treks´-ate) (MTX), 127,
   146, 163
microscope (my´-crow-scope), 65, 66, 71, 85
monocytes (mon´-oh-sites), 32, 69
   immature, 70
monocytic (mon´-oh-sit-ick) leukemia, 56
mouth sores, 127
6-MP (6-mercaptopurine), 147
MTX (methotrexate), 127, 146, 163
murmurs, 26, 27
muscles, 16
myeloblasts (my-ell´-oh-blasts), 60
myelocytes (my-ell´-oh-sites), 70
myelogenous (my-ell-odge´-in-us) leukemia, 56
myelomonocytic (my´-ell-oh-mon-oh-sit´-ick)
   leukemia, 56

N

nausea, 128, 172
needles, 65, 80
negative RBCs, 184
nerves, 18
nervous system, 18
neutrophils (new´-trow-fills), 69
nonlymphocytic leukemia, 56
normal values, 67, 68

nuclear explosion, radiation and, 47
nucleus (new´-klee-us), cell, 7
nurses, 118

O

"on a protocol," 87
"on study," 87
oncogenes (ahnk´-oh-jeans), 45, 46
oncologists (ahnk-kah´-la-jists), radiation, 173
Oncovin (ahnk´-ko-vin) (vincristine), 126, 140
ondansetron (Zofran), 128
organ systems, 10-20
organs, 10-20
oxygen, 13, 24, 26, 156

P

pain, bone, 111
papilledema (pap-ill-id-deem´-ah), 110
parents, 123
pathology (path-ah´-la-gee), 5
PEG, 144-145
periwinkle plant, 140
petechiae (peh-tee´-key-eye), 28
physiology (fizzy-ah´-la-gee), 5
plasma (plaz´-mah), 23, 24, 28
platelet count, 105
platelet transfusion, 105, 186
platelets (plate´-lets), 23, 24, 28-29, 30, 36, 37,
   38, 68, 71, 103, 178
"playroom people," 119
Pneumocystis (new-mow-sis´-tuss), 106
polio, 202
port, 155-162
positive RBCs, 184
prednisone (pred´-nih-zone) (PRED), 110, 126,
   127, 142-143, 163
"prepped," 79
prick, blood tests and, 65
progranulocytes (pro-gran´-you-low-sites), 70
progranulocytic (pro-gran-you-low-sit´-ick)
   leukemia, 56
prolymphocytes (pro-lim´-foe-sites), 70
promonocytes (pro-mah´-no-sites), 70
"protocols" (pro´-toe-calls), 87
psychiatrists, 119
psychologists, 119
pulse, 20
Purinethol, 147

R

radiation (ray-dee-ay´-shun), 47
   cranial, 170, 173-174, 176
   craniospinal, 171, 174
radiation oncologists, 173
radiation therapy, 47, 111, 113, 137, 169-176
radiotherapists, 173
RBCs (erythrocytes; red blood cells), 21-22,
   24, 26, 28, 30, 36, 37, 38, 68, 103, 156,
   178, 184